Praise for *The Vitality*

'Full of science and statistics, this self-help book explains why such basics as good sleep, daily movement and a good diet have such a huge effect on health across the spectrum.' – **LARISSA NOLAN**

'It's full of great practical advice.' – **BRENDAN O'CONNOR**

'His passion for a lifestyle-based approach to human health shines through.' – **PAT KENNY**

'The heart of the book [is] a plea to make that new start, at any stage of life.' – **EMILY HOURICAN**

'It's a must-read.' – **JOE FINNEGAN**

'Two of the big takeaways from the book are, firstly, how uplifting it is and, secondly, how easy the book makes it to start these changes.' – **JENNIFER MCSHANE**

'This book really makes an impression on you but is very easy to read and understand.' – ***ALIVE AND KICKING*, NEWSTALK**

Things your future self will thank you for

DR MARK ROWE has been a practising family physician for 30 years and is the founder of the award-winning Waterford Health Park. As the first medical doctor in Ireland to be certified in lifestyle medicine, Mark is passionate about shifting the mindset from simply a 'pill for every ill' to encouraging people to be more active participants in their own wellbeing, preventing burnout and enabling you to live better for longer.

His TEDx talk 'The Doctor of the Future: Prescribing Lifestyle as Medicine' has over 100,000 views. During the pandemic, he started a popular well-being podcast, *In The Doctor's Chair*. You can learn more about Mark and his work at www.drmarkrowe.com. *Things Your Future Self Will Thank You For* is his fourth book.

Things your future self will thank you for

Small changes, lasting results

Dr Mark Rowe

Gill Books

Gill Books
Hume Avenue
Park West
Dublin 12
www.gillbooks.ie

Gill Books is an imprint of M.H. Gill and Co.

978 18045 8232 9

Design by iota (iota-books.ie)
Print origination by Sarah McCoy
Edited by Kerri Ward
Printed and bound in Great Britain by Clays Ltd, Elcograf S.p.A.
This book is typeset in Quixote Regular.

Dr Mark Rowe uses the medium of story regularly to convey important messages about health, hope and healing. Any resemblance to any person, living or deceased, is entirely coincidental. This book is not intended as a substitute for the medical advice of a physician. The reader should consult a doctor or mental health professional if they feel it necessary.

The paper used in this book comes from the wood pulp of sustainably managed forests.

A CIP catalogue record for this book is available from the British Library.

5 4 3 2 1

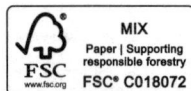

MIX
Paper | Supporting
responsible forestry
FSC
www.fsc.org   FSC® C018072

This book is dedicated to you, the reader,

As your future unfolds one breath,

one step and one day at a time,

May you find purpose and peace,

May you find strength and serenity,

May you find wisdom in valuing your wellbeing,

May you never stop learning,

growing and starting.

To your future.

CONTENTS

Your Personal Fulfilment

Your Relationship with Self and Others

Introduction:

Say Hello to Future You

The past is in your
head, let it go.
The present is in your
heart, let it flow.
The future is in your
hands, make it grow.

Allow me to reintroduce you to an important idea, something I'm sure you intuitively know: you're not the same person you were ten years ago, five years ago or even last year. You've changed physically, psychologically and probably personality-wise too. Your tastes and personal preferences are likely different, and you may no longer want or like the same things. And that's OK. In fact, it's more than OK – it's the reality of who you are at this moment. From your metabolism and mindset to your health and happiness, the only constant in life is constant change. Everything and everyone is changing, whether you sign up for it or not.

A story from Greek mythology that illustrates this idea perfectly is the 'paradox of the ship of Theseus'. It poses an interesting question that has puzzled even the most eminent of philosophers.

Theseus was a hero known for slaying a monster known as the Minotaur. Legend has it that when Theseus returned to Athens after slaying the Minotaur, his ship was given pride of place in the harbour there as a permanent reminder of his tremendous achievement. Each year subsequently, his brave voyage was reenacted. As the years passed, pieces of his ship, which was made entirely from wood, naturally began to weather and decay. In turn, each piece of wood that rotted was repaired and eventually replaced by a new plank, until the time came when every single original piece of wood in Theseus' ship had been replaced. This raises the question – was it still the ship of Theseus, or was it a different ship? If it was different, then at what point in the repair process did it cease to be the original ship? Or was it still the same ship of Theseus by virtue of its function? Did the essence of the ship remain the same despite the frequent changes?

Now let's extend this concept to your human body. Just like the ship of Theseus, your cells and body are part of a continuum of constant change.

Your body contains over 30 trillion cells with a daily turnover of around 330 billion cells, as older cells die and are replaced by newer ones. The vast majority of these are red and white blood cells, which live between several days and a few months, followed by cells that line the gut wall. Every 80–100 days, 30 trillion cells will have been replaced in your body – the equivalent of a brand-new you! There are also trillions of bacteria – collectively known as the microbiome – living in your intestines which weigh in at several hundred grams and replace themselves frequently.

Just like Theseus' ship, you too are constantly changing. As well as the inner architecture of your cells, your thoughts and beliefs, attitudes and behaviours may well be changing every day. How you look and appear to the outside world is also changing in terms of how you are biologically 'ageing' – something that is influenced by a wide range of factors. Are you then still the same person if all your cells are different? Is your identity purely physical or do you have an essence that remains unchanged?

Take a moment to recognise just how much you have changed and grown in the past 10 years. What might be different about you now compared to then? How have you changed in attitude, outlook and perspective? What has enabled you to become the person you are today? What about the person you will be in 10 years' time? What might have changed then?

In his TED Talk, 'The Psychology of Your Future Self'[1], Harvard psychologist Dr Daniel Gilbert brilliantly describes the 'end of history illusion' – the false belief that who you are now is who you will always be. His research has found that we greatly underestimate how much our values and personality traits are going to change in the next 10 years. This bias in terms of how you see yourself can have negative consequences for decision-making for the future, as you have difficulty imagining that, one day, you will no longer be the current version of yourself. It is so much easier for your brain to salute your life journey up to now, acknowledging the growth you have experienced and real changes you have made, than it is to imagine any future changes you might make. So, while you readily perceive that you are not the same person you were 10 years ago, you are unlikely to see the next 10 years through the same lens.

A sentiment that I have heard over the years from some of my older patients is 'If I had known that I was going to live this long, I'd have taken much better care of myself along the way.' That's one of my motivations for writing this book – that you are encouraged and empowered to take action now so you don't experience those same regrets in your future and, more importantly, so you can reap the rewards of longer-term improved health and wellbeing. Staying independent, living your best life on your own terms in your own way, pursuing your dreams, living your purpose.

My own purpose is to continue to spread the message of positive health and 'lifestyle medicine' interventions in three ways:

Firstly, and most importantly, to encourage and support people like you to become more active participants in your own wellbeing, and in doing so be an advocate and a positive example for others to emulate.

Secondly, to encourage physicians and healthcare professionals to see things differently and to add more of these evidence-based tools to their own toolkit of treatment options to support people to get better and stay well.

Thirdly, through an appreciation that actions speak louder than words, to continue to deepen and further develop my own understanding of wellbeing practices. It's all about progress, a commitment to 'never stop starting'.

Many times over the years, I have seen patients whose tentative plans of becoming healthier have been derailed by feelings of overwhelm and decision fatigue. We are generally not good at appreciating the cumulative benefits that can result from the consistent application of small, positive changes. Often this type of change is incremental, happening in seemingly imperceptible ways. Knowing this, how then to plan for the future? Simply start with the reality of who you are right now. Adding or subtracting very small things to or from your life while leveraging the benefits of time can make a real difference to your lived experience. Who you become in the future depends on your choices today.

A metaphor for change that I often use with my patients in my consultation room is the traffic light model.

Red represents something you commit to stop doing. Perhaps no longer bringing your mobile phone to bed, eating late at night or procrastinating.

Orange is a reminder of the many positive health habits in your life already. Many people take their strengths for granted and forget their existing positive lifestyle practices, whether that's spending time with their friends, walking regularly or reading.

Green represents one very small positive change you could make to enhance your wellbeing and vitality. Perhaps starting to add more colour to your food choices, ending your morning shower with 15 seconds of cold water or listening to the birds singing as you sip your morning coffee outdoors.

This book is not another quick-fix solution to transform your life. You won't find any fad diets or magical manifestations in its pages, nor will you be encouraged to undertake a gruelling marathon towards an impossible destination of perfection. Instead, *Things Your Future Self Will Thank You For* is about the reality of YOU, right here, right now, with all the messy imperfections of your past and present life circumstances. It is about accepting today's reality as a starting point to inch forward, slowly but steadily. It is about embracing the daily commitment of consciously choosing to take good care of yourself and the people that matter to you.

The Butterfly Effect is the idea that a tiny change in one part of a system can have a huge impact elsewhere – how a metaphorical butterfly beating its wings in Brazil could cause a tornado in Texas. In the same way, one small positive change you bring into your life today could make an enormous difference to your future vitality. Everything is interconnected.

At the start of the book you will find a chapter on the science of habit formation and solid strategies to successfully build and maintain positive changes. The rest of the book is then divided into four separate sections: things for physical health and wellbeing; things for emotional wellbeing; things that foster personal fulfilment; and things that strengthen relationships.

In these four sections you will find a menu of ideas and sustainable self-care strategies to enhance the wellbeing of your current and future self, such as embracing exercise as medicine, minimising ultra-processed food, unplugging in nature, building a sense of purpose, practising self-compassion and many more small, positive shifts you can undertake. Simply try one of the suggestions for a period of time, observe what happens and then decide whether or not to continue with the experiment or embark on a new one. Using both the scientific evidence (the why) and the support strategies (the how), you can build the bridge to lasting positive change.

By understanding future you more clearly in terms of your goals, dreams and aspirations you can work towards a healthier tomorrow while reducing the negative impact of life's stressors today.

The American speaker and author Earl Nightingale once said to 'never give up on your dream just because of the time it will take to accomplish it. The time will pass anyway.' Of course, none of us can turn back the clock and start again, but starting today can create a brand-new ending. To paraphrase the Danish philosopher Kierkegaard, life can only be understood looking back, but it must be lived and experienced by looking forward. As you look forward to your future, let your choices and decisions be guided by those things that you will thank yourself for. This can lead towards a better relationship with future you; not perfect, but perhaps 1 per cent wiser, stronger, healthier, happier and more hopeful. Your future self starts today.

Small Steps To Future You

Let me live by the art of small steps.

Finding the courage to face my fears.

Knowing that action speaks louder than words.

Valuing the difference between empty promises and
everyday efforts.

Staying curious, open in heart, spirit and mind.

Listening carefully when wise voices proffer truth and
good advice.

Being patient, knowing that many problems solve
themselves.

Being persistent, appreciating the value of progress.

Being present to each unfolding experience, allowing
future me to emerge.

Recognising that life's challenges and setbacks are simply
signposts along the way, supporting me to become
wiser, stronger and better.

Enabling me to never stop learning, growing and starting.

Inching forward:

One day

One step

One breath at a time

Living by the art of small steps

Becoming my best future self.

Leverage the science of habits

Building new habits can take a lot longer than the quick-fix formulas often advertised. Research from University College London shows that it takes between 18 and 236 days – 66 days on average – to reach a stage where it becomes easier to keep going with your new habit than to let go of it.[1] That's 66 days of committing to exercise even when you feel you're too tired or too busy or it's wet and windy outside.

Habits are hardwired, automatic and ritualised behaviours that shape your health and life overall. You make your habits and then your habits make you. Over time, the meals you order, the exercise you take and the work habits you cultivate all add up to influence the person you become. As a creature of habit, you tend to keep thinking, feeling and doing what you have always thought, felt and done. In fact, research has found that more than 40 per cent of the actions people performed each day weren't actually conscious decisions, but habitual behaviours carried out while the participants were thinking of something else.[2]

As a doctor, I can appreciate just how difficult positive change can be, even when we understand the benefits of making the change in question. Many people know what they *should* do in terms of their health, but they stay chained to their existing habits. I call this the intention gap, the very real gap between who you are today as you read this and future you with new habits firmly ingrained.

The basal ganglia are very old brain structures located deep in the brain tissue near the skull base. They play a key role in in the coordination of complex movement patterns such as grasping, walking and eating, and along with the executive lobe, they help the brain prioritise the rapid deployment of a particular pattern of movement. Speed of response was vital in a world where potential danger lurked beyond every bush. This automation is also key to forming habits. Being able to automate a behaviour pattern through the basal ganglia also means you do not have to use your willpower muscle to consciously choose and carry out an action. This consumes valuable brain energy – something that is always in relatively short supply! Instead, you can simply 'replay' the desired behaviour – for example, brushing your teeth or locking your front door – without giving it much thought.

At the beginning of a habitual activity such as brushing your teeth, some nerve cells or neurons in the basal ganglia activate and 'fire', then remain quiet during the activity itself before firing again at the end. This conserves brain energy and also allows you the freedom to think about something else throughout the automated task.[3]

You may have believed that creating a new habit is all about willpower, but in fact this isn't the case. This is because willpower is essentially a muscle in the brain that becomes depleted with usage. The more actions you are able to automate by turning them into a habit, the more energy you will have to devote to other tasks at work or at home. Building a new habit in essence is all about building new pathways in your brain and reinforcing those new brain connections repeatedly; over time, these thread-like connections are strengthened, turning into metaphorical steel cables of a hardwired habit. This is why successful behaviour change and habit formation is less about willpower and much more about the 'skill power' of habit automation.

Successfully building a new habit into your life can be incredibly rewarding and fulfilling. You are more likely to succeed if you follow some or all of these guiding principles:

Start on the inside

All sustainable change happens twice: firstly on the inside, then again later when it shows up in your outer life. The challenge is to join the dots, connecting how you think and feel with what you do and how you behave. Ask yourself, why is it important for you to build this new habit? What's motivating you to build this new habit? How confident are you of succeeding? What value will this new habit bring to your life?

Values are part of who you are and are powerful levers to support positive change. They provide the 'why' – compelling reasons to take action. For example, the habit of volunteering connects with the value of kindness, exercise connects with the value of health, keeping a written journal connects with the value of personal growth and so on. And as they say, if you know your why, the how gets easier.

Connect your habit with future you

Think of a change or habit you'd benefit from making right now, something your future self would thank you for. Imagine the benefits of bringing this new habit into your life and how something might change for the better as a result; for example, volunteering may bring new friendships and social connections, while reading and self-development could expand your world view.

Now visualise a future version of yourself who has adopted these habits and create a contrast in your mind between this future you and your current lived reality. Awareness of this gap can support you to take action to begin to close it, starting today. Similarly, visualising yourself in old age looking back at today allows you the opportunity to thank your current self for the choices you are making and think about how proud and satisfied you will one day be because of them.

Recognise the reward

One of the key drivers for both positive and negative habits is the reinforcement provided by reward. At a biochemical level, reward releases dopamine, one of the brain's favourite feel-good chemicals. Dopamine is released in the brain's limbic system, which connects with the basal ganglia. Because of this, habits executed through the basal ganglia can become reinforced with positive feelings and emotions, making these habits more memorable.

This is why it is helpful to focus on the rewards you will reap from building a new habit. In the case of taking exercise, this would mean focusing not only on the longer-term objective benefits of improved health, but more immediately the feel-good factor of more energy, relief from stress and an uplift in mood.

Recognise the trigger

It's important to understand what the trigger of a given behaviour is, particularly in the case of a habit you wish to break. Let's say, for example, that you comfort eat late at night while watching Netflix because you feel bored or stressed. Doing this gives you the reward of distraction or temporary stress relief. Avoiding the trigger for a while (in this case, watching Netflix) and choosing to read instead may prevent the negative behaviour (comfort eating).

Design a 'Ulysses Contract'

One of the major challenges in building a bridge to future you is transcending the powerful gravitational pull of the present – what's happening today, right now. The architecture of the human brain is designed for fear detection and survival, which too often makes the future a prisoner of the present moment. When faced with the competing choice of something good now or something potentially better in the future, your brain's decision-making is skewed towards the now. This is one reason why it can be so easy to make choices that feel good in the present moment, but that have negative consequences later on. This is where designing a 'Ulysses Contract' can help.

Thousands of years ago, having been a triumphant leader in the Trojan war, Ulysses was embarking on his long voyage home by sea. While plotting his course, he realised that his ship would pass an island where many beautiful Sirens lived – women who were famous for singing melodious songs that so completely enchanted sailors, they would run aground on the rocks trying to get closer to them.

While Ulysses was curious to hear the songs for himself, he didn't want to endanger his crew. His problem wasn't the present, rational Ulysses but instead the future, illogical Ulysses – the person he knew he would become when the Sirens came within earshot. So he hatched a plan. Ulysses ordered his men to tie him securely to the mast of the ship, to fill their ears with beeswax and ignore any of his pleas to release him. This way, he was able to return home safely without being fatally derailed.

So many things impact the choices we make every day, from our immediate context to the influence of others. Most of us are very poor at anticipating in moments of cool deliberation how differently we may feel in a given situation in the future. Designing your present environment so that future you doesn't deviate inadvertently from your 'plan' can protect your willpower and help you better navigate any unexpected events that may influence your decisions. For instance, filling your fridge and cupboard with healthy foods makes it so much easier to eat well when you are feeling tired or stressed and may be tempted to order a takeaway. Taking social media apps off your phone can prevent mindless scrolling when boredom hits. Arranging a strength-training session early on a Saturday morning with friends is a good way to get you to bed early the night before.

A Ulysses Contract is a win-win deal that makes room at the inn for future you, despite competing and often conflicting choices. Without compromising your values or exhausting your willpower, it enables you to behave in closer alignment to the person you want to become.

Change one habit at a time

Many people overestimate what they can achieve in one year but underestimate what they can achieve in five!

It's easy to fall into the trap of trying to change too much, too quickly, and to overestimate the role that willpower plays in habit formation. Changing a habit isn't easy and consumes a lot of mental energy. Focus on one habit at a time, and once that new behaviour pattern has become habitualised and established, then you will have the mental energy to work on another. Willpower is always in limited supply, and it's weakened throughout the day by the myriad everyday choices and temptations we face, as well as being further depleted by emotional stress, poor quality nutrition and suboptimal sleep. Willpower is strongest in the early part of the day, which is why it is often most effective to schedule new habit changes in that window. If you want to strengthen your willpower, then exercise, mindful meditation and high-quality brain nutrition (like nuts, seeds, oily fish, berries, dark greens, etc.) can help.

Try habit stacking

Consider stacking positive change onto something else you are already doing. For example, if you want to do more exercise, consider doing some squats while brushing your teeth or engaging in social activities that involve more movement, such as hiking or dancing.

Practise affirmation

Writing a regular positive affirmation is another way to support future you. Expressing your affirmations in the present tense brings the future into the present moment. I believe you are far more likely to persist with a habit that you frame positively and specifically, like eating a rainbow of colour or walking 10,000 steps a day, than one you frame negatively, like eating fewer unhealthy snacks or feeling less stressed. If you believe that you are running away from something, then you will always feel like something is chasing you!

SOME IDEAS FOR POSITIVE AFFIRMATIONS

- I am living my values
- I am grateful for all my blessings
- I am always learning
- I value the gift of my life
- I cherish my relationships
- I follow my dreams
- I breathe consciously and clearly
- I let my actions speak louder than my words
- I never stop starting
- I am, I can and I will!

Find your tribe of support

Who can support, strengthen and encourage you? Who can become an accountability partner for your habit change? Conversely, who are the energy vampires that you might need to avoid? The people you spend time with have a big influence on your habits, for better and for worse. The 'mirror neurons' in your brain mean you tend to adopt the habits, attitudes and mannerisms of the people you spend the most time with right throughout your life – not just when you are a teenager!

If you spend time with people who eat healthily and exercise regularly, you're more likely to eat healthily and exercise regularly as well. If you spend a lot of time with people with less-than-healthy lifestyle habits, chances are that you're going to adopt those unhealthy habits too.

Start small

You've heard the old adage that an elephant is eaten one bite at a time. Effective change takes time and continuous effort. It is so easy to become frustrated, disillusioned and dejected at your apparent lack of progress, not to mind the off days and inevitable slip-ups. Which is why there is so much upside potential in starting small – really small. While committing to completely overhauling your diet may leave you feeling overwhelmed, adding a single serving of nuts or seeds to your breakfast every morning could feel much more achievable while also moving you towards your ultimate goal.

Small shifts in the mind, body, heart or spirit can produce profound healing over time. A great question to ask yourself is 'What's the smallest change that can provide you with evidence that you're moving in the direction of the person you want to become?'

Aim for progress, not perfection

Many attempts at positive change tend to fail after an initial 'honeymoon period' of a week or two when you revert to type. A written journal can be invaluable here, to track days and times when things went well and, perhaps more usefully, those days and times when your intentions didn't go as planned. It is so important to get back on track again as soon as you can after the inevitable blip or speed bump. Reflecting on your lived experiences each week is a great opportunity to learn and grow, and it may help you gain some insight into how you can stop self-sabotaging. What excuses will you no longer accept? What can become better and how can you achieve that? What gets measured gets improved!

Celebrate your wins

It is crucial to reward yourself for small 'micro-wins' along the way, to celebrate your success, reinforce your efforts and recognise forward momentum gained. Reward yourself often – you deserve it!

Who will you be in five years' time if you keep doing what you're doing right now? Apply this question to your health, your relationships, your career, your goals and your personal development. What habits could you build or break, starting today, that could open up new possibilities in your life? Answering this question is the key to unlocking the potential of future you.

Your Physical Health and Wellbeing

Don't take your health for granted today, or you'll spend your tomorrows trying to get it back.

Become the CEO of your own health

When did you last have a medical check-up? How much do you understand about your family medical history? Do you know the key numbers when it comes to your blood pressure, blood sugar, cholesterol and so on? What's one small step you can take today to improve your 'health IQ'?

As a GP, I'm well aware that many people have a blind spot when it comes to their basic health data – things like family history, blood pressure and cholesterol. There are several important numbers when it comes to your long-term health. Knowing your body and knowing these numbers means that you will notice changes and get new symptoms checked out as they arise. I call this 'being the CEO of your own health'.

Ask the CEO of any organisation about their roles and responsibilities and they will likely describe leadership, strategic planning, decision-making, governance and operational oversight in many areas. These include establishing the organisation's vision and goals and ensuring accountability by monitoring key performance indicators while taking appropriate action to ensure that the agreed strategies are implemented. They will identify risks and threats to this success and have contingency plans in place that balance short-term performance with longer-term, sustainable growth.

No matter what your profession or primary role is right now, you can appoint yourself today as the CEO of your own health.

When you become the CEO of your own health, you take charge of your most priceless asset and deepen your understanding of all its facets. You become crystal clear on your values and vision for your current and future health plans, making informed decisions about your everyday health choices and investing in sustainable habits that align with your personalised plan. You seek expert advice as needed and invest wisely in appropriate resources – from appointing an expert mentor or coach to availing of a gym membership to learning new skills, like strength training or how to cook healthy meals. You schedule timely health check-ups and screenings, mindful of your personal and family history. You know the key performance indicators that keep you on track. As any CEO will tell you, the numbers matter – what gets measured gets done! All this knowledge becomes power, enabling you to take your head out of the sand and take action – just like Joe did.

I'll never forget the day Joe first walked into my consulting room. His wife Mary had booked the appointment to discuss her own health issues, and asked if he could attend the consultation with her. I had never met Joe before and, like many 45-year-old men, he rarely attended the doctor (later, I learned that Joe had only ever been in the practice once, more than 20 years earlier, when a nasty dog bite to his leg had necessitated a tetanus injection and some stitches).

After a while it became clear that there were issues between Joe and Mary, and things became quite heated. One minute, Mary was talking about her sleep issues and the next she digressed into how uncommunicative Joe had become at home and how she felt he wasn't coping with the stress he was under. His workplace was closing and, having worked there for close to 25 years, Joe would soon be unemployed for the first time in his life. At first Joe denied this vehemently, but Mary persisted and Joe became visibly angry. His voice became agitated as he spoke about how no one understood the pressure he was under. All of a sudden, Joe's speech was slightly slurred and he became less coherent.

'My arm and face feel funny,' he managed to say.

A quick examination revealed his blood pressure to be very high at 180/100 with a fast, thready pulse. Neurologically he had altered sensation and slight weakness in his left facial muscles and left arm. My strong index of suspicion was an early evolving stroke, so we arranged for Joe's immediate transfer to hospital by ambulance for urgent further evaluation.

The next time I saw Joe was just after he was discharged from hospital a week later. He had been lucky. He had suffered a mini-stroke (also known as a TIA, or 'transient ischaemic attack') and had made a full recovery. The source of his troubles lay hidden away under the bonnet, undetected for many years. Tests revealed that Joe had high blood pressure, raised 'Non-HDL' cholesterol and blood fat, and borderline blood sugar (HbA1C). Combined with a waist circumference of 44 inches, a sedentary lifestyle and stress levels that were through the roof, Joe was a ticking time bomb waiting to explode.

That was more than two years ago.

Since then, Joe has turned his life around, becoming an active participant in his own health journey. He now has regular blood tests and full check-ups. As part of our preventative care programme, he gets a 24-hour blood pressure monitor at least once a year to ensure optimal blood pressure control. His father and uncle had both developed bowel cancer in their 50s, so Joe opted to undergo a screening colonoscopy which picked up polyps on his bowel wall. These are potentially harmful if left undetected as they can eventually become cancerous, but their early discovery meant they could be removed before that happened. He has been prescribed several medications to optimise cholesterol and blood pressure and to thin the blood, all of which he is taking fastidiously. As a result of other positive health changes, the doses of some of these have already been significantly reduced.

Joe has now developed a great health IQ, a term I use to describe having the right knowledge, awareness and attitude to make informed choices that support your long-term health and wellbeing. Here are the main ingredients in improving your own health IQ:

First, know yourself. This may sound facile but believe me, many people (especially, but not only, men) can stick their heads in the sand and ignore important symptoms for months or even years before taking appropriate action. Appreciate what's normal for you (think bowels, waterworks, energy, sleep, mood and mental health) and get things checked out if you notice a change from your usual pattern. Get to grips with your family medical history and avail of a regular preventative check-up with your doctor.

Having a good family doctor is important too. Modern healthcare can be lifesaving, but it's extremely siloed with many different 'ologists': the skin doctor (dermatologist), eye doctor (ophthalmologist), heart doctor (cardiologist) and so on. None of these doctors looks at the overall person the way the family doctor does, seeing you in the context of your family and community, translating and putting together all the different parts of the puzzle. We are all unique in our own way and having someone who can support you in your healthcare journey can be invaluable.

Of course, the numbers and health IQ are just one part of it. Here are some of the other things Joe did to become the CEO of his own health.

Over a period of several months, Joe went from being sedentary to embracing the 'exercise as medicine' prescription. He incorporated 30 minutes of brisk walking each day as well as strength training in a supervised class twice a week. Regarding his food choices, he pivoted from being an ultra-processed food junkie to eating lots of 'real food'. While he still allows himself a treat, much more of his food intake now comprises vegetables, fruit, pulses, whole grains, nuts and seeds. He keeps his penchant for red wine now to a glass or two at weekends. No radical changes, just a gradual evolution in awareness allied to positive action.

Not only did Joe begin living a healthier lifestyle in terms of nutrition and exercise, but he has also learned to manage stress. He learned the importance of resting and recharging, reducing his work commitments and saying no when needed. He committed to a wind-down every night and began to really value his sleep routine. As a result, he felt that his stress levels had come down, which improved his decision-making (especially when it came to craving sugary snacks!).

He began to value his relationships too by making more time for friends. He has gone on several weekend hikes with friends as he has rediscovered the wellbeing benefits of time in nature.

Each of us is unique, so your precise prescription for health improvement is unique to you. There is no 'one size fits all'. What was key for Joe was that he understood the interconnected nature of the many aspects to his health and wellbeing. He learned that there was no point focusing just on his dietary habits if he didn't also address his stress levels or his sleep. He focused on feeling good, finding fulfilment and having fun. He adopted a sustainable lifestyle plan that moved him forward towards more positive health. These gradual improvements bedded in as habits over a two-year period. The benefits for Joe are not just enhanced energy and feeling much fitter in the short term, but a significantly altered trajectory of his health in the long term.

To become the CEO of your own health, my suggestion is that you start thinking about your health as an investment asset. We all know that investing in pensions, property, portfolios of stocks and plain old-fashioned saving plans will produce returns over time and can provide greater financial freedom and security.

Important as this is, the benefits of investing in your health are far, far greater. Investing today will ultimately lead to an increase in what is called your 'healthspan', or the number of years you stay healthy and free of disease or disability, as well as your lifespan (with the usual proviso of 'lady luck'!). Furthermore, this increased healthspan provides a second 'return on investment' as you will have more time to create memories, enjoy experiences and build relationships. Of course, having some financial resources and the great health to enjoy them is a double bonus, but without health, money is meaningless.

Rome wasn't built in a day and no one should ever believe that significant, sustainable change happens overnight. However, what *can* change today is your commitment to being a more active participant in your own wellbeing. While informed financial advisors can support your investment decisions and financial health, so too can an experienced health professional leverage your health IQ to help you become the CEO of your own health.

Begin to make smart, strategic decisions that support consistent health gains. It will pay rich dividends now and into your future. Start today – it only takes one small step.

Below are some of the important numbers to be aware of when it comes to your long-term health – the key components of your health IQ. Some of these can be easily checked by you at home – for example, belly circumference with a tape measure, and pulse and blood pressure with easily accessible home devices. I encourage you as the CEO of your own health to be on the front foot, as it were, and discuss the tests mentioned with your doctor. As you know, what gets measured gets managed. This is why it can be so helpful to schedule a doctor's visit when you are well, in order to proactively plan relevant and timely tests.

Body mass index

Body mass index, or BMI, is a well-known measurement derived from weight in relation to height. BMI categories include underweight, normal weight, overweight, moderately obese and severely obese; for example, a BMI of between 25 and 30 falls in the overweight category, while obesity is determined by a BMI of over 30. There are several online calculators you can use to find your BMI measurement.

While higher BMIs are associated with adverse health outcomes, BMI does not take account of your body composition (how much of your body weight is made up of muscle versus fat) or where in your body your fat is stored. While BMI can give a helpful guide, fat stores and muscle mass are far more important, which is why your belly size measurement can be much more relevant to your health.

Belly size

The extra pounds that midlife can bring tend to accumulate around the belly area and are known as visceral fat. Visceral fat is belly fat that is found deep inside the abdomen, in the spaces between the abdominal organs and in tissue called the omentum. Visceral fat is different to subcutaneous fat (fat found just beneath the skin) and it can have significant downsides, putting you at increased risk of heart disease, high blood pressure, diabetes and other metabolic conditions, osteoarthritis, sleep apnoea, gallstones, fatty liver and even dementia.

You can measure your belly size quite easily using a tape measure. With your belly relaxed, measure the circumference at the level of the belly button. This is not the same as your trouser size. For men, belly size should be less than 40 inches (102cm), and for women it should be less than 35 inches (89cm). Larger measurements indicate excess belly fat, and an increased risk of health problems.

Blood pressure

Your heart is like a muscular pump, and every time it contracts it generates a pressure in your blood vessels known as systolic blood pressure. In between each contraction the heart relaxes, and this pressure is known as diastolic blood pressure. Blood pressure is therefore denoted by two separate numbers, with normal blood pressure typically around 120/80mmHg (mmHg stands for 'millimetres of mercury', and it's the conventional way of measuring blood pressure).

Without getting your blood pressure checked, there is no way of knowing whether it's normal or not. Raised blood pressure is a silent condition and the first 'symptom' of it may be a life-threatening complication, like Joe's mini-stroke. More insidiously, raised blood pressure can affect vision and kidney function and is a significant factor in memory loss from vascular dementia.

High blood pressure is very common in Ireland, with research from The Irish Longitudinal Study on Ageing (TILDA) suggesting two-thirds of people aged over 50 have it.

Welsh GP Dr Julian Tudor-Hart, also known as the 'father of high blood pressure', famously described his 'rule of halves': he found that only half of all people with high blood pressure know about it, only half of those people get it treated, and only half of those have it properly controlled. In other words, the vast majority of those with raised blood pressure don't have it optimally managed – perhaps as few as one in eight.

Target blood pressure should in general be as close to 120 systolic as possible (perhaps a little higher for older people). For every 20mmHg increase in systolic blood pressure or 10mmHg increase in diastolic blood pressure, the risk of dying from a heart attack or stroke doubles.[1]

The SPRINT trial was carried out on a group of adults aged 50 or older who had systolic blood pressures of at least 130 in addition to other risk factors for heart disease. It found that participants achieving a lower blood pressure of under 120 reduced their rate of cardiovascular events by 25 per cent and reduced the overall risk of death by 27 per cent. This equated to living for an estimated extra three years, evidence that knowing your numbers matters![2]

Many people feel anxious when attending the doctor and this 'white coat effect' can cause blood pressure to temporarily rise. The best way to check your blood pressure is with a 24-hour blood pressure monitor, which is the gold standard. Failing that, you can learn to check it yourself regularly at home and bring the readings to your doctor.

Blood sugar

A haemoglobin A1C (HbA1C) test is a blood test that measures what your average blood sugar (glucose) level was over the previous 90 days.

HbA1C can be an excellent way to identify insulin resistance and diagnose type 2 diabetes or pre-diabetes in the absence of typical symptoms (such as fatigue, thirst, etc.). Normal levels of HbA1C are under 42, while levels of between 42 and 48 are considered pre-diabetes and over 48 indicates diabetes. There has been an explosion in the number of people with type 2 diabetes in recent years and knowing your HbA1C levels enables you to take positive lifestyle changes to prevent, reverse or better manage type 2 diabetes.

Blood lipids

Elevated cholesterol is a major risk factor for heart disease in both men and women. Traditional measurements included total cholesterol (normally under 5), LDL (under 3), HDL (over 1) and triglycerides (under 2). Lower levels may be recommended depending on your personal medical and family history. More recently, 'non-HDL' is considered the best measure of cholesterol. A normal level of non-HDL cholesterol is under 3.8. A 40-year-old male with a non-HDL cholesterol of 5 and without any other risk factors for heart disease has a 23 per cent chance of a major cardiovascular event, such as a heart attack, by age 75. This can be reduced to less than 4 per cent by lowering non-HDL cholesterol by 50 per cent. Just another example of why numbers matter![3]

ApoB is an important protein found in LDL cholesterol that helps to clear cholesterol from the blood. With a normal range of under 100, it provides a direct measure of atherogenic particles, with higher levels associated with heart disease and stroke. Positive lifestyle changes can help reduce it.

Lipoprotein (a), also known as Lp(a) for short, is much more 'sticky' than LDL cholesterol. High levels of Lp(a) can clog up your artery walls, leading to heart disease or stroke at an earlier age. It is a significant inherited risk for heart disease and is also thought to increase the development of blood clots. You should consider getting this checked at least once in your lifetime, especially if you have a family history of heart disease or stroke.

Pulse

An irregular pulse – also known as atrial fibrillation – is a major cause of stroke, particularly in older people. Knowing how to check your pulse rate and rhythm is an important part of self-care. With your hand extended and wrist slightly bent, use the second and third fingers of your other hand to feel your pulse at the level of the wrist, behind the base of your thumb. Calculate the rate by counting it for 10 seconds, then multiply by six to give the pulse rate per minute. The average pulse rate is about 70 beats per minute for a healthy adult, while lower levels (up to a point!) can signify enhanced fitness. The rhythm of the pulse should be regular; if it is irregular or there are 'skipped beats', you should see your doctor.

Prostate

While a detailed description of the various bodily systems and their functions is beyond the scope of this book, many men remain ignorant of the importance of the prostate gland. A small organ about the size of a walnut, it normally increases in size by about one to two per cent a year from age 40 onwards. The urethra passes through the middle of it, which is why an enlarging prostate can cause waterworks symptoms such as urinating more often, change in the urine stream, urinating more at night, etc.

A blood test known as the PSA test, along with a prostate exam, can provide additional insight into whether such symptoms may indicate prostate enlargement or early prostate cancer. When it comes to your prostate, if in doubt, check it out!

Finally, as you begin working to improve your health IQ, a word of caution. Increasingly people are using wearable technology to measure all sorts of health data. From heart rate variability both at rest and with exercise, to blood pressure, steps taken and calories burned, these can all provide helpful metrics to support you as health CEO. As we know, what gets measured gets managed. The flip side of this 'quantified self' is potential health anxiety for some. There's always a balance to be struck. Own your health data, but don't let it own you.

Eat fewer
ultra-processed foods

Beekeeping has become a very popular pastime in recent years, and I am fortunate to have some special friends and patients who gift me occasional jars of locally produced honey. It's so interesting how wild honey can vary so much in both taste and texture. Of course, bees are wonderful creatures, and not just in terms of their honey-making ability; they play a pivotal role in the pollination of plants and supporting our environment. The political makeup of the hive, with the queen and her worker bees, is also fascinating. While worker bees and the queen share identical genes, the queen lives much longer. Compared to the worker bees who feed on pollen, the queen's lifestyle habits are very different; as well as being cared for continuously, she gets to eat royal jelly which is predigested for her by her attendant bees. A terrific symbol of how good food can positively impact health and longevity.

Unfortunately, this idea is far removed from the everyday lived reality of so many. One of the hallmarks of the modern Western diet is the amount of ultra-processed food (UPFs) eaten each day. Think fast food, fizzy drinks, protein bars and, indeed, pretty much anything out of a packet or wrapper. Consumption of UPFs represents up to 80 per cent of total caloric intake in adults aged over 18 in the US and Canada, with confectionery and sugar-sweetened beverages being the most consumed items.[1] Now comprehensive research published in the *British Medical Journal*[2] has strongly linked high intake of these foods to more than 30 separate negative health impacts – including a 50 per cent increase in both anxiety and heart disease, increased rates of depression and other common mental health disorders, sleep issues, increased risk of diabetes and all-cause mortality. In one study, after 18 years of follow-up, each additional daily serving of UPF was associated with a 7 per cent increased risk of heart disease.[3]

There's no doubt that the modern, highly processed diet contains far too much sugar. According to the National Cancer Institute in the United States, the average American adult or child consumes about 17 teaspoons of added sugar a day. This equates to 68 grams or about 270 calories.[4] This compounds to 60 pounds of added sugar consumed per year, more than 2 to 3 times the recommended amount for men and women respectively. The American Heart Association recommends that men should consume no more than nine teaspoons (36 grams or 150 calories) of added sugar per day. Women should consume no more than six teaspoons (25 grams or 100 calories) per day.

Processed foods such as fizzy drinks, biscuits, cakes, 'low fat' yogurts, sweets and desserts are all high in added sugar, but there are also many hidden sources – think cereals, bread, soup, gravy, processed meats and even marinara sauce! Hidden sugars are present in the following ingredients commonly found in ultra-processed foods: high-fructose corn syrup, corn sweetener, brown sugar, malt sugar, molasses, fruit juice concentrates and additives ending in 'ose', such as sucrose, maltose, lactose, glucose, fructose and dextrose. And then there is the more obvious white sugar that is spooned into many cups of coffee and tea. All that excess added sugar can create a cascade of negative consequences for your health as it is broken down through the liver, which can become over-whelmed, eventually leading to fatty liver. This, along with cellular inflammation and raised blood pressure, increases your risk of heart disease and stroke.

Excess sugar can be 'addictive' in that sugar releases dopamine, a brain neurochemical involved in pleasure and reward. While your blood sugar initially goes up, giving you a 'sugar high', insulin release then brings the blood sugar level back down. This causes your blood sugar to 'yo-yo', leading to feelings of irritability as you crave more sugar to get the level back up. This can play havoc with your mental health. In terms of mood, I see added sugar being the source of feelings of stress and anxiety, even though many people will turn to sugar for comfort and relief when feeling stressed. It's a case of one step forward and three steps back.

The potential adverse effects of excess sugar consumption include weight gain and increased visceral fat stores, joint pain and inflammation and type 2 diabetes as your pancreas 'burns out' from overwork. Advanced glycation end products (AGEs) are harmful compounds formed when sugar combines with protein or fat in the bloodstream through a process called glycation. At high levels, AGEs can increase the risk of many diseases, while also damaging collagen and elastin in the skin, leading to skin ageing. Finally, excess sugar can accelerate biological ageing, leading to memory loss and cognitive decline.

Of course, cutting down on excess sugar consumption isn't always easy. It was a big challenge for Tony, a patient of mine who worked long hours as a truck driver. Aged

49 and naturally tall and slim, he had been an infrequent attender for most of his adult life. So when he came in one day for a routine check-up, I was surprised to see how much he had changed. Tony had gained a substantial amount of weight, evidenced by his increased belly size of 43 inches. Tests revealed that his blood fat, cholesterol and sugar levels were all raised, and his blood pressure was borderline. Tony had developed a strong sweet tooth, eating several bars of chocolate a day and washing them down with lots of sugary drinks. He felt that the sugar kept him going during long drives, and a bar of chocolate was always easy to find at a pitstop. What had started as an occasional treat while he was on the road had become his way of life.

With a strong family history of heart disease, Tony wanted to find out how he could improve his health status. Less than two years later, Tony had transformed himself. His blood pressure and biochemistry were back to normal, and his belly size was back down to 38 inches.

When I asked him how he had done it, Tony explained, 'That day a couple of years ago was a real wake-up call, and I realised that I was harming my health so much. It was all about habits really. Now I'm moving a lot more every day, and I prepack healthy food and water before any of my trips. I never stop at a garage when I'm hungry now – the temptation to buy chocolate was just too much before, especially when I was tired.'

So, what to do in a world with so much sugar and so many ultra-processed food options? It starts with awareness! Now that you know more about the potential downsides, you can decide for yourself if you would like to do something about it. If so, then perhaps try some of these strategies.

Keep a food diary

Keeping track of what you are eating, when and why provides a realistic overview of your current habits. Patients often find this helpful as recording your complete eating and drinking habits for a week or two – including weekends! – provides a benchmark against which to measure change. I encourage recording the times at which you eat (to measure your eating window), your mood when you eat (to check for emotional eating and impact of stress) and any other associations that arise (for example the impact of eating out or seeing advertisements for food).

Once you get to grips with your current reality, a question to consider is 'What would eating more healthily look like for me? What are small, sustainable changes I could make to achieve this?' Reviewing your progress regularly – ideally once a week – is a key part of this exercise, so you can see the times, days and places when things went according to plan, and also when they didn't. Regularly reviewing what went well and what could improve can provide you with a basis for longer-term sustainable, positive change as it serves to remind us that nobody (including you!) is perfect and that eating more mindfully is a lifetime commitment to valuing your health, as opposed to a short-term fad of dietary restriction.

Learn the language of labels

Become a detective when you are shopping and learn to read food labels - you might be surprised just how much hidden added sugar is in some of your choices. Consider some healthy swaps: perhaps oats with ground seeds and nuts instead of regular box cereal; natural yogurt with berries instead of sugar-loaded flavoured yogurts; extra virgin olive oil and balsamic vinegar instead of sweetened salad dressings. When it comes to the bittersweet truth of sugar and your health, it's very much a case of less is more!

Be more Mediterranean

Science shows that the Mediterranean diet can support more positive mental health, increased healthspan and longevity, with a significant reduction in heart disease, stroke and other chronic health conditions.[5,6] As a diet of inclusion it remains flexible, with the focus on eating a rainbow of colour and consistently taking in nutrients, as opposed to the number of calories consumed: think plenty of fruit and vegetables, whole grains, extra virgin olive oil, beans, peas, lentils, oily fish, nuts, seeds, herbs and spices. It also emphasises a restricted eating window of a maximum of 12 hours, moderate portion sizes and avoiding snacking in between meals.

While it might be easy to describe a 'perfect' diet and nutrient intake, real life isn't perfect for any of us, nor will it likely ever be. So, based on your current circumstances and lived reality, what might an improved, healthier version of your dietary habits look like for you? Perhaps more colour, more seeds or an extra portion of vegetables?

Take the Socrates test

Socrates once wrote that before you let words out of your mouth, ensure they pass through three gates – are they true, are they necessary and are they kind? Similarly, before you let food into your mouth, see if it passes through the three same gates of truth, necessity and kindness. Firstly, is what you are about to eat 'true' food? Is it real food and wholesome, or is it ultra-processed? Secondly, is eating this food necessary? Are you eating because you feel hungry or to fuel your body, or eating because you feel stressed, upset or simply bored? Finally, is eating this food kind? Is it kind to your body and all its organs, kind to your brain and memory, kind to the trillions of cells that work so hard to support your health and wellbeing? Is it kind to the planet in terms of sustainability?

Reevaluating your food choices through these three gates will move you closer, day by day, to the idea of food as medicine, helping to nourish your mind, body and soul.

Take cold showers and hot saunas

Greek physician Hippocrates may well have been onto something all those centuries ago when he prescribed cold baths as a remedy for fatigue. In Roman times, visitors of bath houses traditionally rotated through a number of heated rooms and pools and ended with a dip in cold water. This ritual of the 'frigidarium', or cold plunge, is something that has persisted in many spas and saunas worldwide. When I think of cold showers, my mind harks back to my school days when the mandatory showers after physical education class were always cold – ice cold, as I remember them. Cold enough to put you off cold

showers for life! Nowadays, year-round sea swimming
has become a cultural phenomenon here in Ireland. Many
people I know rave about the sea dip for its feel-good
benefits, considering it a non-negotiable part of their self-
care routine, even in the depths of winter. This has made
me curious to delve into the science a little bit more.

Hormesis is an adaptive response of the body to a
low-grade temporary stressor. It provides benefits in
supporting the body against future stressors. It may
strengthen cells' repair mechanisms, increasing their resilience and boosting their ability to survive. Because your
skin has far more cold than heat temperature receptors,
cold exposure through having a cold shower (between 10
and 15 degrees Celsius) can be a highly effective form of
hormesis. It activates the sympathetic nervous system and
its physiological fight-or-flight response. Blood pressure
increases as vessels near the skin surface contract, with
blood then being diverted towards the vital organs as
the body works to protect them via the 'stress response'.
Afterwards this process is reversed as the body warms
itself up again, a process which may improve circulation
to and from muscles. This temperature and blood pressure change leads to electrical impulses travelling from
nerve endings in the skin to sensory areas of the brain.
As a result, you get a welcome boost in neurochemicals
including noradrenaline and endorphins.

Endorphins stimulate opioid receptors to act as 'natural painkillers' which can make you feel more calm, energised and optimistic. They dampen down the impact of stress while inducing a positive feeling similar to the 'runner's high' (but without the running!). As one of the key chemicals that triggers the fight-or-flight response, noradrenaline increases blood pressure, heart rate and the functioning of large muscle groups, including their blood flow and ability to contract. It is one of those 'super chemicals' that supports early morning alertness, focus and concentration, responsiveness to pain, mood, memory and your degree of interest in things. It can enhance the performance of cells in the brain and most bodily organs and can also lead to an improvement in mood and overall feelings of wellbeing.

Cold therapy may also support the body in producing mitochondria. Mitochondria are the magical, energy-producing parts of your cells. More mitochondria means an improved metabolism, which can lower cellular inflammation and may reduce the risk of developing many chronic health conditions – think heart disease and diabetes for starters. This may also help with weight control as an improved metabolism leads to more energy and more calories being burned.

So what do the studies show? Research from Norway published in the *International Journal of Circumpolar Health* strongly supports the use of cold-water immersion for both physical and mental health benefits. Researchers found that men who regularly participated in cold-water immersion overall had lower visceral fat and boosted brown fat production.[1] The main function of brown fat in the body is to increase your metabolism to produce and help the body retain heat. Brown fat also has a higher concentration of mitochondria than regular fatty tissue, and it can help prevent heart disease, diabetes and obesity.

Additional research from the Netherlands involving more than 3,000 study participants found that ending a warm shower with a cold shower led to a 29 per cent reduction in self-reported sick leave, even when the cold shower lasted for as little as 30 seconds. While the 'cold shower brigade' still complained of ailments like everyone else, they were able to keep going without needing to take time off. A comparison with regular exercisers found that exercisers reduced their sick leave by 35 per cent, whereas those who took both exercise and regular cold showers reduced their sick leave by 54 per cent! While the exact reason for this remains unknown, these numbers suggest that cold showers may give an immune system boost, helping the body to combat viruses and stay healthier. And as if that wasn't enough, more than 60 per cent of the study participants chose to continue their cold shower habit after the 90-day study concluded because they had enjoyed the wellbeing boost it gave them so much.[2]

Now, I'm not suggesting that it will be nice! Cold-water exposure can be uncomfortable, especially at the beginning, as it stimulates pain receptors. And before you go switching up your shower routine, there are a few important caveats to be aware of here. Firstly, remember that you are not a polar bear; cold exposure is a shock to the system. Sudden exposure to severe cold could potentially adversely shock the body or trigger a cardiac event including an arrhythmia (heart rhythm disturbance) or heart attack. If you have heart disease or a circulatory condition, talk to your doctor about whether cold therapy is something you should avoid or be cautious about. Be cautious about how long you expose yourself to cold water, remembering that you will lose body heat up to 25 times faster in cold water than you would at the same ambient air temperature. Just a few minutes of cold-water exposure can trigger hypothermia with serious attendant health risks.

My advice is to start slowly, perhaps by finishing your regular shower with 15 seconds of cold water. Gradually build up the duration by 15 seconds a week until you are having a 2-minute cold shower after eight weeks. Finally, only consider cold-water swimming after receiving the green light from your doctor and after properly acclimatising.

Overall, a cold shower can be a wonderful morning ritual to build self-discipline, grit and resilience, raising your stress threshold and possibly even bringing other psychological benefits such as a reduced tendency to procrastinate. It's a reminder that you have the power to choose small, actionable steps each day that enable you to live with more vitality and provides a 'daily reset', a way of stepping out of your comfort zone. In addition, a cold shower can lead to lower water consumption and a saving on your energy bills, making it good for the planet as well as your pocket! So why not give it a try?

POTENTIAL BENEFITS OF A COLD SHOWER
- Increases your stress threshold
- Provides a thermoregulatory workout
- Increases brown fat production
- Improves metabolism
- Strengthens immune system
- Improves circulation
- Lowers inflammation
- Increases pain threshold
- Builds willpower, grit and resilience
- Boosts mood and mental wellbeing
- Increases energy and vitality

Saunas have been widely used in Finland for thousands of years. One in every three Finns uses them – and their usage doesn't signify an affluent lifestyle. Culturally speaking, the Finnish sauna represents a stress-free zone, a gathering space to relax and recharge.

Research from Finland highlights the benefits of regular sauna usage in significantly reducing risk of heart disease, high blood pressure, stroke, memory conditions and even premature death. They are also associated with a reduced risk of many other common health conditions, including chest conditions such as asthma, COPD and pneumonia.

A study carried out by the University of Eastern Finland followed 2300 men aged 42–60 over a period of 20 years. The researchers found that increased frequency of sauna use led to a reduced risk of fatal cardiovascular disease, even after allowing for age, lifestyle and other cardiovascular risk factors. Each sauna visit lasted on average 14 minutes at 80 degrees Celsius. Men who used the sauna between four and seven times a week were 63 per cent less likely to experience sudden cardiac death and 50 per cent less likely to die from heart disease. They were also 65 per cent less likely to develop dementia and about 40 per cent less likely to die prematurely from all causes. Those participants who used the sauna two to three times weekly were 22 per cent less likely to experience sudden cardiac death and 20 per cent less likely to get dementia.

Frequent saunas were also associated with lower death rates from stroke and a lower risk of high blood pressure.[3]

A sauna provides brief exposure to extreme heat which increases the body's core temperature and results in a mild hyperthermia. Just as with cold showers, having a sauna is a form of hormesis, as a low-grade temporary stress exposure that triggers a cellular repair response. Heat exposure also leads to increased levels of substances known as heat shock proteins, which play a role in repairing cells damaged by stress. In the environment of the warm sauna, blood vessels near the skin surface widen, which increases blood flow through them and helps to cool the body. This increases heart rate, improves overall blood flow and is thought to improve the health of the lining of the blood vessels themselves (known as the endothelium). An important measure of inflammation in the body known as CRP also lowers with sauna usage in a direct, dose-dependent manner.

In a way, the sauna simulates a form of low-grade cardiovascular exercise. Cardiac output – a measure of the amount of work done by the heart in response to the body's need for oxygen – increases significantly as blood flow is diverted from the body's core to the skin to enable sweating and cooling. This can be significant, with up to a pint of sweat being lost during a short sauna session! Just like exercise, saunas increase something called BDNF, or brain-derived neurotropic factor, which is involved with the development of new cells in areas of the brain linked to memory, learning and cognitive function (the hippocampus and cerebral cortex). This may explain why Finnish research has found a significant reduction in the risk of developing Alzheimer's disease amongst those who used a sauna at least three times a week.

Saunas can be very good for your mental health too, increasing both noradrenaline and endorphins in much the same way as cold showers and bringing all the same mood and focus-boosting benefits. As a mindful practice, saunas have been associated with a reduced tendency to depression.

Of course, nothing suits everyone and common sense is important. Especially if you have a heart or other health condition, it's important that you talk to your doctor first before using saunas. Saunas can trigger dehydration and low blood pressure. Be careful not to overdo it – start with 5–10 minutes and gradually build time, as tolerated, up to 20 minutes. Drink plenty of fluids (non-alcoholic!) before-hand and take electrolytes afterwards to rehydrate. Always avoid saunas if you feel unwell. Taking exercise before or during a sauna may trigger a heart arrhythmia, clot, low blood pressure or severe dehydration and must be avoided.

Overall, the science of saunas suggests significant potential health benefits. Stay biologically younger, increase your healthspan and delay the physical and mental manifestations of ageing. Support more positive mental health and enhance your overall wellbeing, all while recharging from stress in a pleasant and health-enhancing environment. Something to think about introducing as part of your wellness routine. Your future self may be glad you did.

Enjoy great coffee

Legend has it that coffee was originally discovered by a goat herder known as Kaldi in Ethiopia, whose goats became energetic and sleep-averse after eating the berries of the coffee tree. Kaldi informed the abbot of the local monastery, who made a drink with the berries and discovered that it kept him awake and alert through the long hours of evening prayer. The abbot shared his discovery with the other monks at the monastery, and word of these energising berries spread across the world, leading to coffee cultivation and trade.

For many people, one of life's simple pleasures is a perfect cup of coffee, while the flavoursome aromas and feel-good factor are enhanced exponentially when enjoyed in good company. Think of how many great conversations have taken place over a coffee cup.

Back in medical school, coffee was a staple of the last-minute cramming sessions that exams brought. For over-worked and stressed junior doctors, caffeine was a late-night essential, helping to keep the bleary-eyed awake through the small hours on call. It was functional and freely available, but that was about it, really. No amazing aromas or fulsome flavours, the coffee we drank then was more chicory than chic!

Fast forward 40 years and there has been an explosion of interest in coffee and all its varieties. Furthermore, coffee is now understood to have a variety of potential health benefits.

Coffee contains B vitamins, magnesium and polyphenols, which have antioxidant properties that can reduce inflammation and oxidative stress. In fact, coffee beans contain over 100 biologically active compounds which can boost metabolism, improve insulin sensitivity and lower cellular inflammation and oxidative stress. Perhaps it is these antioxidant polyphenols in coffee that provide the greatest health-boosting benefits. These substances help to negate the oxidative stress in the body caused by ageing and lifestyle factors and environmental toxins.[1]

A review of coffee, caffeine and health in the *New England Journal of Medicine* has highlighted how moderate coffee consumption of no more than four cups a day consistently correlates with a reduced risk of several chronic health conditions.[2] In the Nurses' Health Study, which involved more than 83,000 women, drinking four cups of regular coffee a day was associated with a 20 per cent reduced risk of stroke. An 11 per cent reduction was also seen in drinkers of decaffeinated coffee, implying that the benefits may relate to specific ingredients in the coffee rather than the caffeine per se. A meta-analysis of 36 studies in men and women found a 15 per cent reduction in cardiac mortality, heart disease, stroke and heart failure in those who consumed no more than four cups of coffee a day, compared to those who drank no coffee. Further research that analysed death from chronic health conditions found that moderate coffee intake reduced the risk of deaths from cardiovascular diseases by 21 per cent, compared to non-coffee-drinkers.[3,4]

Coffee could also lower your risk of developing type 2 diabetes; that's what a meta-analysis involving more than 45,000 people has found. The research, which followed participants for more than 20 years, found an inverse association between the amount of coffee consumed and the risk of developing diabetes: compared to no coffee consumption, six cups of coffee a day reduced the risk by 33 per cent.[5] On top of that, research also connects coffee consumption with reduced risk of gallstones and Parkinson's disease.

Of course, coffee contains caffeine, a stimulant that is potentially addictive. Too much caffeine can cause insomnia, anxiety and irritability, while sudden withdrawal from caffeine can trigger low mood, fatigue, headache, and anxiety. At higher doses of consumption (generally over 300 mg), caffeine commonly causes negative health effects including irritability, anxiety, restlessness, increased heart rate and unwanted heart palpitations.

Indeed, like many things purported to be 'good' for you, more is not always better. The Interstroke study was a major research project on stroke that involved almost 27,000 people from 32 countries. Recent analysis of this data by researchers at McMaster University in Canada and the University of Galway has found that drinking more than four cups of coffee per day raises one's chances of having a first stroke by 37 per cent. On the other hand, they found that less than four cups daily was not associated with an increased risk of stroke.[6]

Having said all that, there is some evidence that coffee can be good for your mental health and wellbeing. A meta-analysis of studies involving more than 330,000 participants found a 28 per cent reduced risk of depression in those who consumed the most coffee compared to the least. Furthermore, they found the greatest benefit, or 'sweet spot', seemed to occur with caffeine intake up to about 500 mg per day – or about four cups of coffee.[7]

You might consider sharing a cup with your garden plants too, given that coffee grounds are rich in nitrogen and small measurable amounts of potassium and magnesium, both plant nutrients. It also helps attract microorganisms to support plant growth while improving water retention, drainage, and aeration of the soil.

Some of the more recent insights into coffee consumption concern its timing. Coffee promotes alertness by blocking adenosine receptors, adenosine being an inhibitory neurotransmitter which tends to suppress arousal and promote sleep. By delaying your first coffee until you have been awake for 90 minutes or so, adenosine levels will have risen while cortisol levels will have fallen, thereby optimising the feelings of being alert and awake after your morning coffee.

Caffeine can reduce total sleep time, increase the time it takes to fall asleep and worsen perceived sleep quality. It can take 8 hours to wear off, so mid- and late-afternoon coffee can certainly keep you awake at night. In fact, the half-life of caffeine is 4–6 hours, meaning that 300 milligrams of caffeine in your eleven o'clock Americano may result in at least 75 milligrams of caffeine circulating in your blood 12 hours later. You don't have to be a maths genius to figure out why too much coffee can keep you awake!

If you typically reach for a cup of coffee first thing upon waking, you may want to try waiting a little while. Cortisol, the stress hormone, is generally at its highest first thing in the morning, while adenosine is at its lowest. Drinking coffee shortly after waking can increase the chances of feeling jittery and anxious instead of experiencing a boost in mood, motivation and attention. Furthermore, early morning coffee can trigger a significant rise in your blood sugar and increased tolerance to caffeine, meaning you may need more to experience the same effect. The research suggests that it is far better to wait until a couple of hours after waking, when cortisol levels are dropping and adenosine levels are rising. Coffee at this stage will provide a far better feeling of attentive alertness and avoids the potential cortisol-assisted jitters from drinking it earlier in the morning.

While caffeine is a mild diuretic, the water in coffee more than counterbalances this; therefore, drinking coffee counts towards your daily fluid intake. Furthermore, research from Nottingham University has shown that drinking coffee can stimulate brown fat production, which burns calories by generating heat.[8] So drinking coffee may help you lower your overall fat stores – provided, of course, you consider what you put into it! Calorie-laden cream and sugar certainly won't add anything to the list of coffee's potential health benefits.

Of course, like everything, there is no one-size-fits-all. While many people thrive on caffeine, feeling alert and better able to focus after a cup of coffee, some people are exceptionally sensitive to the stimulant effects of it even at low doses. Genetic factors play a role here and older adults may also be more sensitive to its effects. Some people are simply faster metabolisers of caffeine and clear it from their systems more quickly. As we are all different, it's important that you know yourself well enough to appreciate just how coffee and caffeine impact how you feel. This is especially important if you are suffering from anxiety, toxic stress or sleep issues.

If you are sensitive to caffeine, try decaffeinated varieties and you may experience similar health benefits. And while I love to savour and enjoy a cup or two of really good coffee, I suggest avoiding caffeine in the second half of the day to support your sleep. If you have difficulty sleeping, cutting it out for a while can be very helpful.

Overall, habitual coffee drinking can be good for your health – not just reducing your risk of heart disease and diabetes, but increasing alertness and attentiveness, which can support you to live a longer, healthier life.

If coffee is not your thing, then perhaps drink tea. Green tea especially is rich in polyphenols, especially flavonoids.

The fermentation process used to make green tea boosts polyphenol levels significantly higher than in black or red teas. These polyphenols may help slow the effects of ageing on the brain. Green tea also contains L-theanine – an amino acid that increases brain 'relaxation chemicals' such as gamma-aminobutyric acid (GABA), serotonin and dopamine.

Two studies from the Harvard School of Public Health, involving both men and women working in healthcare, have associated tea drinking with a reduced risk of diabetes over a long duration. Drinking two to three cups daily may also reduce the risk of heart disease, stroke and premature death.[9]

While drinking tea appears to be associated with better health, it's difficult to know whether the tea itself is the answer. Perhaps tea drinkers simply live healthier lifestyles. In either case, if you like tea – especially green tea – drink it to enjoy it and your future self may reap health benefits as well. A toast to your health!

Move as if your life depends on it

Have you taken any exercise yet today? If not, can you put this book down right now and move for just a few minutes? Something as simple as climbing five flights of stairs a day can lower your risk of heart attack by up to 20 per cent![1] Every little counts.

When I went to medical school in Dublin back in the 1980s, the number of lectures and tutorials we got about exercise was precisely nil. None! There wasn't so much as a mention of the health-enhancing and mood-boosting benefits. In hindsight, I believe this was partly because the medical model at that time emphasised treating illness through medication and/or surgical intervention. But I also believe that as a profession that was somewhat inaccessible to the average person in terms of methodology and language, and with a significant power dynamic between the doctor and the patient, medicine traditionally had a certain 'mystique'. Would the idea of prescribing something as straightforward as exercise be seen as worthy of all that training and expertise?

Having said that, there were a few notable exceptions. The late Professor Risteárd Mulcahy, an eminent cardiologist, espoused exercise through his own everyday actions. Professor Mulcahy was considered something of a revolutionary, banning smoking in cardiac wards in St Vincent's University Hospital in 1970 and becoming a founder member of the Irish Heart Foundation in 1966. Tall and thin as a rake, and an avid squash player well into his 60s and beyond, I vividly remember one interaction with him when I was a medical student. I was strolling along the footpath with a classmate outside St Vincent's Hospital when we heard someone approaching quickly from behind. As he overtook us, we realised it was Professor Mulcahy walking at an extremely brisk pace. We would have had to jog just to keep up with him! Similarly, our professor of surgery used to run up several flights of stairs during ward rounds with his large team of junior doctors and medical students in tow, trying to keep up with him. As students we saw this simply as eccentricity, something we might have had a laugh about when safely out of earshot, but in hindsight it's clear to me now that they both knew something about the health benefits of exercise. Of course, they were right. Exercise and movement is the 'greatest pill of all' and can do more to optimise the healthspan and wellbeing of future you than anything else I know.

Movement is medicine, and science is beginning to comprehend the vast interconnected web of biochemical and molecular signalling that enables exercise to provide substantial health-enhancing benefits. These include a dialling-up of cell integrity and repair systems and corresponding dialling-down of cellular inflammation.

Research by Stanford scientist John Ioannidis has compared the benefits of taking medication to exercise for the secondary prevention of chronic health conditions. Secondary prevention refers to early detection of a disease and treatments that prevent it from getting worse. The study found that exercise either exceeded or matched medication for the secondary prevention of coronary heart disease, stroke and pre-diabetes (the exception was heart failure, where medication did outweigh exercise).[2] I mention this study not to dismiss the benefits that medication can bring, but to highlight the tremendous potential benefits that can accrue from taking regular exercise. Commit to taking just

90 minutes of exercise over the entire week, and you can reduce your risk of dying from all causes by 14 per cent. Compared with being sedentary, taking regular exercise can add up to a decade to your life expectancy.

Committing to persistent action means not just starting but restarting after every slip-up and bad day (or week, or month). It also means avoiding the pursuit of 'all or nothing' perfection. When Niamh attended my practice, she had been experiencing high levels of stress – particularly in her work life, where she was a very successful senior corporate executive. There had been considerable flux in her global team with consistently increasing expectations. The impact on Niamh was a textbook reaction to chronic stress: as she experienced more and more stress, she stopped exercising and abandoned the self-care habits that had helped her to be at her best for so long. My firm belief is that those who don't make time for exercise eventually make time for illness.

'I just don't have time for exercise,' responded Niamh to my gentle enquiry about her exercise habits. Something I have found helpful over the years is to reframe this idea by turning it into a positive. What's the smallest step you can take to provide you with evidence that you are literally moving forward? It's all about baby steps. In Niamh's case, it was about trying to incorporate 'micromoments' of movement.

'Would you be able to exercise for five minutes each morning?' I asked.

'Don't be ridiculous,' Niamh answered. 'Of course I would.'

So that became the goal. First thing each morning, Niamh put on her running shoes and walked or jogged for 5 minutes. When I saw Niamh again six weeks later, she felt much better.

'Your suggestion of five minutes first thing each morning has really helped,' she told me. 'Five minutes is such a short period of time that I couldn't not agree to it. That would have seemed ridiculous. It was easy to achieve, and accomplishing it felt surprisingly good from a self-worth point of view.'

At my suggestion, Niamh had also kept a written journal through this time, as expressive writing can provide significant clarity and act as a catalyst to embed positive changes. She shared with me what she wrote about this positive change she had made:

'I felt that I was taking back control of my morning, my day and ultimately my life. In some ways, Dr Mark's task was too easy for me – but that was the whole point, I suppose. It stopped me from the negative cycle of self-recrimination at not having time to go to the gym or work out "properly".'

'After a couple of weeks I started exercising for longer, increasing to 10, 20 and gradually to 30 minutes most mornings. It felt like a good thing to do. I followed Dr Mark's suggestion carefully, though, to always do the five minutes. Even on my busiest days, or days when I felt tired or fed up, five minutes became my non-negotiable habit. I've always been someone who is 'all or nothing'. Great at exercising for a while, then doing little or none for months at a time. Fooling myself that if I didn't have an hour to go to the gym, then I didn't have time for exercise. That was how I saw things in the past. But I can honestly say that this simple mindset change had changed my life for the better.'

So, when it comes to movement as medicine, here are some suggestions to consider in support of future you.

Move more – every step counts

Research carried out in 2022 examined the daily step counts and health outcomes of a nationally representative sample of American adults aged 40 years and older. Compared with taking just 4,000 steps per day, taking progressively more steps per day was significantly associated with a reduction in mortality, with the lowest death rates noted in those who walked more than 12,000 steps daily. There appears to be a direct relationship between higher step counts and reduced deaths from cancer, heart disease and all-cause mortality.[3] In addition, research carried out in 2012 has found that briskly walking for 450 minutes each week is associated with living around 4.5 years longer than doing no leisure-time exercise.[4] While this data is observational, and not evidence of causation, it certainly points firmly in the direction that when it comes to your long-term health, more steps are better.

Move smarter – the magic of 'Zone 2' training

If you can talk forever while exercising, then the workout is termed Zone 1, whereas if you are struggling to finish a sentence then you are in Zone 3 or higher. Zone 2 is that sweet spot of pushing yourself gently beyond the comfort zone of chatty conversation, while exercising. Being able to talk but not sing while exercising, while not feeling inclined to have a conversation, is the upper level of Zone 2 training. Zone 2 training generally falls between 60 and 70 per cent of your age-adjusted maximum heart rate, which is often a slower heart rate than many people are accustomed to exercising at.

For example, if you are 50 years old, you can calculate your Zone 2 heart rate using the following formula: 220 – your age (50) = 170 (maximum heart rate). 60–70 per cent of 170 = 102–119 bpm.

If you are less fit, you may enter Zone 2 at a lower heart rate.

The American College of Lifestyle Medicine recommends at least 150 minutes of this form of exercise per week. This type of training is incredibly beneficial to fat-burning in the shorter term as it supports mitochondrial health. Mitochondria are the 'batteries' of your cells and have the capacity and metabolic flexibility to burn both glucose and fat as fuel. In Zone 2 training, fat is primarily the fuel source and using fuel in this way builds significant stamina and endurance. If you are not fit, however, your exercise capacity will be limited by your ability to burn glucose as fuel. This has the downside of creating lactic acid, leading to cramp and limiting capacity to exercise. Zone 2 training builds a foundation of fitness and endurance that keeps lactate levels below the point of accumulation, or less than 2 millimoles per litre.

While the rate of perceived exertion – also known as the 'talk test' – is a good approximation of Zone 2 training, you can fine-tune this further by checking your lactate level while exercising. This can be done at a sports medicine facility or by yourself with a handheld device. The goal is to ensure the lactate level remains below 2 millimoles while exercising. If it rises above 2 at a low level of exercise, this means you are metabolically unfit.

The good news is that it's really easy to exercise at the Zone 2 level. Think brisk walking or walking uphill, using the elliptical machine or exercise bike, swimming or playing tennis. Aim to build this up to 45 minutes, four times a week, over time and you will make yourself physically and metabolically so much fitter over time, boosting longer-term healthspan while supporting longevity.

Move faster – boost your VO_2 max

VO_2 max is a measure of the amount of oxygen that your body can consume per kilogram of body weight per minute. The fitter you are, the higher your VO_2 max will be. While originally thought to be only of value to high-performance athletes, it is now recognised as being highly relevant for the healthspan and longevity of even non-athletes.

Increasing your VO_2 max requires you to exercise at your maximum level of exertion, so talk to your doctor first to ensure that it is medically suitable for you. Having warmed up, exercise for 4 minutes at the maximal pace you can exert for the entire 4 minutes. Then exercise gently for 4 minutes, allowing your heart rate to reduce back to below 100 beats per minute. Repeat this process four times in total, followed by a warm-down and a good stretch. Doing this once or twice a week is more than enough to support long-term improvements in VO_2 max. The higher your VO_2 max, the greater your chances of living a healthier life for longer. A study that reviewed the health data of 750,000 veterans aged between 30 and 95 found that extremely high aerobic fitness was associated with the greatest survival and that cardiorespiratory fitness was inversely correlated with long-term mortality.[5] The bottom line is that your degree of fitness matters big time.

Don't settle for being average. If you want to be an above-average 90-year-old, then you don't want to be an average 60-year-old. My recommendation is to go to a professional laboratory and have your VO_2 max checked.

Move for better balance – take the one-leg standing test

Balance exercises just don't feature in common conversation, which is a real pity because the science is unequivocal: better balance helps prevent falls and all the associated comorbidities. What's more, balance issues are common and a major cause of disability as you age. When it comes to your balance, it's very much a case of 'use it or lose it' as, once lost, it's hard to regain.

In fact, your balance is a powerful prognosticator of how long and healthily you will likely live. Research published in the *British Medical Journal* measured several thousand 53-year-old men and women using three tests: the one-leg standing test, grip strength and how quickly they could stand up from a seated position. Thirteen years later they were remeasured. The one-leg standing test provided the strongest correlation with longevity, as those participants who could stand for longer than 10 seconds were three times less likely to have died than those who lasted 2 seconds or less. Overall, the study found robust associations between standing balance time, chair rise speed and grip strength at age 53 and all-cause mortality rates over 13 years of follow-up. [6]

The one-leg standing test is something you can easily do yourself at home. Remove your shoes and, with your hands on your hips, simply stand on one leg and time yourself. The test finishes when you put the raised foot down on the ground or move the planted foot. Do the best of three attempts to get your average time. Repeat on the other side.

Now repeat the test with your eyes closed. This makes it much more difficult as your brain has to work harder to stay balanced using two other important sensory systems: firstly, the vestibular system in your inner ear; and secondly, proprioceptors in your muscles that provide feedback loops to the brain.

ONE-LEG STANDING TEST: TARGET SCORES PER AGE CATEGORY
Under 40: 45 seconds with eyes open,
15 seconds with eyes closed.

Aged 40-49: 42 seconds with eyes open,
13 seconds with eyes closed.
Aged 50-59: 41 seconds with eyes open,
8 seconds with eyes closed.
Aged 60-69: 32 seconds with eyes open,
4 seconds with eyes closed.
Aged 70-79: 22 seconds with eyes open,
3 seconds with eyes closed.

Great ways to improve your balance include integrative exercise such as yoga (by building focused flexibility, mobility and postural strength), Pilates (by supporting a stronger core), and especially tai chi. This gentle form of slow, low-impact rhythmic movements combined with breathing and mindful awareness was originally a martial art. Tai chi has its roots in Taoism, an ancient Chinese philosophy based on opposing forces known as yin and yang. Bringing mind and body into balance through tai chi is thought to promote harmony and health. Studies have found it helpful for balance, flexibility and muscle strength, as well as recharging from stress and reducing blood pressure. As little as eight weeks of tai chi practice can reduce fear of falling and improve balance.

In addition, consider habit stacking balance exercises on top of something you already do – for example, standing on one bent leg while brushing your teeth.

Move for fun – just dance

Dancing is a form of complex movement that can be health-enhancing, social, stress-relieving and fun. It supports a psychological state of flow, as you enter into 'the zone' of being completely energised, focused, absorbed and engaged. Dancing can also improve the workings of your brain and boost memory.

Research published in the *American Journal of Preventive Medicine* in 2016 found that regular dancing was associated with a slightly lower risk of cardiovascular death than regular walking – perhaps due to the stress-busting benefits of social connection combined with the physical exercise.[7] Given the significant positive mental health benefits of listening to music and physical activity, it is not surprising that dance also boosts levels of brain chemicals such as serotonin, enhancing overall wellbeing.

Dancing can make you smarter, too. A 21-year study of people 75 and older published in the *New England Journal of Medicine* examined whether any recreational activities positively impacted mental acuity with ageing, thereby preventing dementia. They found that the only physical activity that protected against dementia was frequent dancing. While doing crossword puzzles at least four times a week reduced the risk of dementia by 47 per cent and reading by 35 per cent, regular dancing reduced risk by a massive 76 per cent.[8] This is because dancing supports neuroplasticity and the development of new brain pathways, thereby building cognitive reserve. Dance also synchronises several brain functions simultaneously – emotional, rational, musical and kinaesthetic – leading to greater complexity of neuronal synapses and increased cognitive acuity. If you're already a regular dancer, this is great news. If not, then it's never too late to check it out.

Move every day – incorporating NEATer movement

Non-Exercise Activity Thermogenesis, or NEAT, is a term used to describe the everyday energy we use when doing everything apart from exercising, sleeping or eating. It is an important and sustainable way to burn more calories and help reduce the risk of chronic cellular inflammation and chronic disease, while also supporting more positive mental health. There are so many ways to bring NEAT into your everyday life. Think household chores (cleaning and cooking), standing more, gardening and walking. This is easily accomplished using simple practical measures such as parking further away from shops or restaurants, getting off the bus one stop before your destination and my personal favourite: the simple act of taking the stairs.

As I pointed out at the start of this chapter, climbing more than five flights of stairs daily can reduce your risk of heart attack by 20 per cent according to recent research from Tulane University.[9]

Whenever I'm at an airport deplaning after a flight, the same choice presents itself. To use the escalator like pretty much everyone else, or to choose the stairway, which is usually wide, inviting and empty. It's interesting just how few people ever use the stairs at the airport (from my own observation, it's less than 1 per cent). I try to ascend those stairs two steps at a time as a reminder that I have agency over my health decisions, a very empowering idea. Making the health-enhancing choice is empowering and enables you to make further positive choices through a sort of upward spiral effect. Now that's 'neat', isn't it?

We can all have peaks and troughs when it comes to any health habit, which is why consistency trumps mountains of motivation each and every time. It's far better to plod along steadily like a tortoise rather than pursue the 'all or nothing' extremism of the hare. Just as Niamh discovered, building the habit of exercise is all about starting. Small, positive changes can compound over time to make a big difference to both the quality of your lived experience and longer-term wellbeing. Every step, every movement and every moment counts.

Be stronger to live better for longer

Imagine yourself at 80 years of age. Will you be able to carry your bag through an airport, even if the wheels fall off it? Will you be able to carry your shopping easily? Will you still be able to bounce up a flight of stairs? If you would like the answer to these questions to be 'yes', then you should start strength training today!

For better and for worse, we are all influenced by the environments we spend our time in. Distraction and temptation can influence our ability to make healthy decisions and derail the very best of intentions. On the other hand, small environmental cues can act as a catalyst for positive change. Which is why I brought a 15kg dumbbell into my office a couple of years ago.

Strategically placed in a prominent position under my desk, the dumbbell is clearly visible to patients. Its purpose is twofold. Partly it is there to remind me about continuing the habit of strength training. We all need reminders! But mainly it serves as a visual prompt for patients to stimulate conversation about this really important health topic. As an experiment it's been really interesting, sparking conversations that actively encourage people to start strength training, while reinforcing the benefits among those (mainly younger guys) who already do it regularly.

Which reminds me of Paul, a patient of mine who visited the practice not too long ago. Glancing at his computer record revealed very little of note. The most recent entry included the results of some standard medical tests several years earlier, all of which were normal. He was on no medication and had no chronic conditions.

When I called Paul into the room, he bounced up from his seat in the waiting area. I asked him about his reason for attendance, and he informed me it was for his driver's licence renewal form. I glanced at my computer screen and had to do a double take – the date of birth put Paul at 83 years old!

'Can you confirm your date of birth again?' I asked, half anticipating an error. But no, it was correct – he had indeed just turned 83. *But biologically, not a day over 70 years*, was what I was thinking as I began to fill the driver's licence form in with Paul observing from a standing position close by.

What happened next, though, left me speechless. Without saying a word, Paul placed his left hand on my desk while he bent in a press-up position to lift the 15kg dumbbell with his right hand. He then proceeded to do a set of dumbbell row exercises, counting each one out loud all the way up to 15.

'Great to see you getting into the weights, Doc,' he said as he stood up afterwards. 'It's something I've been doing myself for years. Swear by it. Keeps me sharp.'

Now imagine yourself at Paul's age. This is not an unlikely scenario given how lifespans have increased in recent decades. Indeed, research from the National Institutes of Health predicts that the number of individuals aged 80 and older by 2050 will have tripled, with more than 447 million worldwide.[1]

Would you like to be still working out regularly then, full of energy and vitality? Still physically strong and functionally independent? Still skiing or playing tennis? Well, why not? It's all about starting. As I read once, if you want to have the things that few others have, you must be willing to do the things that few others will. This quote is so relevant to the health and vitality of your future self.

Stop comparing yourself to the fitness of someone 'your age'. Think yourself younger and make yourself stronger through the regular habit of strength training at every stage of adulthood – even (and especially) 80 years old and beyond. It's not just for boxers or bodybuilders or people who want to look better. Strength training is a key component of staying healthy for men and women alike.

'Stay stronger to live longer' is far from just a catchy soundbite: it's true. And yet while many people walk and move, with a lesser number also taking some aerobic exercise, strength training is a major blind spot for many.[2] Partly perhaps due to its association with a certain 'type' of person – typically the muscle-building gym warrior or elite athlete – many people believe strength training is something that's for 'them', but definitely not for me! Most people simply don't understand what they are missing out on in terms of the health benefits and the longer-term implications for their mobility and functional independence.

As you become older, you start to lose valuable muscle mass. This can be as much as 10 per cent per decade from your forties onwards, with inevitable eventual decline in functional capacity. Not only that, but muscle loss leads to frailty and reduced vitality, which is why a slip or fall in a 70-year-old can so easily result in a fractured hip. It's worth noting that six out of every 10 people who break a hip never fully regain their previous degree of independence. As a result, the simple activities of daily living can become increasingly difficult. Without strength training you are guaranteed to become physically weaker over time, but it doesn't have to be that way. Strength training can reverse this process, keeping you stronger and healthier and lowering your biological age by redefining the conventional concept of 'ageing'.

In terms of your physical health, regular strength training can increase the rate at which you burn calories, also known as metabolic rate, and positively impact body composition by building muscle mass. This improves insulin sensitivity while reducing cellular inflammation and the risk of various chronic health conditions. It can support sounder sleep, and may even be superior to aerobic exercise in terms of providing better sleep benefits.[3]

Recent research published in the *British Journal of Sports Medicine* has found that 30 to 60 minutes of weekly strength training significantly reduced risk of diabetes and heart disease. Specifically, a lowered risk of diabetes by 17 per cent and a 10 to 20 per cent lower mortality from both heart disease and cancer in those who did strength training regularly.[4] A moderate degree of muscular strength is also associated with a 32 per cent lower risk of developing type 2 diabetes in those who are at higher risk of the disease, independent of estimated cardio-respiratory fitness.[5]

Strength training can help reduce blood pressure. It also boosts balance, strength and sense of stability through its positive impacts on bone density, muscle strength and joint mobility. As an important strategy to help offset age-related decline in bone density, it is important in the context of fall prevention and reducing risk of an associated fracture.[6]

Emerging evidence suggests that strength training can be a powerful antidepressant. You were born to move, and the essential purpose of your brain is to enable complex movements as opposed to sitting for too long and (over)thinking. Research shows that strength training supports positive mental health by reducing symptoms of depression and anxiety.[7] It's a wonderful way to blow off steam. It improves mood by elevating mood-boosting neurochemicals and pain-zapping endorphins, increasing feelings of relaxation and reducing stress. Furthermore, endorphins further enhance feelings of positivity, with a mild euphoric feeling experienced at the end of an invigorating strength session. Working towards and achieving goals through strength training, no matter how small those goals are, supports self-confidence and self-efficacy. Overall, it can become a powerful and sustainable form of self-care that supports the mind–body interface.

A study conducted in 2018 which examined the results of 33 randomised clinical trials involving more than 1,800 people concluded that performing resistance training at least twice a week led to a significant reduction in symptoms in people suffering from mild to moderate depression and may be even more effective for those experiencing severe depression.[8]

Scientists in Copenhagen may have discovered why. Recent research has led to the discovery of tiny chemical substances known as myokines which are produced by actively engaged muscles. Myokines are able to enter brain tissue, where they trigger a complex cascade of biological benefits, improving mood, learning, memory and mental health. Indeed, the benefits may be on par with going to therapy or taking antidepressant medication. The myokines produced during strength training can boost brain power overall, building a sharper, more agile and responsive mind. This can build a stronger brain buffer against future memory loss and potential dementia.

Downstairs in the rest of the body, myokines improve the functional capacity of energy-producing mitochondria, the powerhouses or 'batteries' of your cells. Mitochondria convert micronutrients into molecules known as ATP. Strength training is a key way to support mitochondrial numbers and health, thereby increasing your long-term capacity for enhanced energy and vitality.

THE HEALTH BENEFITS OF MYOKINES

- Increase in BDNF = more cells in brain areas vital for memory, learning and higher cognitive functions
- Increase in serotonin = boosted mood
- Increased insulin sensitivity = reduced blood sugar
- Increase in mitochondrial production = enhanced energy
- Increased neurogenesis = more new brain cells
- Increased pain threshold = better pain management
- Reduced cellular inflammation and oxidative stress = slower biological ageing

But there are many different aspects of physical strength – it's not just about how much you can bench press! Recently there is growing understanding of the importance of grip strength as a valid proxy measure for your overall body strength. While being physically stronger supports your living longer, the converse may well also be true. Poor grip strength is associated with accelerated biological ageing. Health risks associated with low grip strength include heart disease, type 2 diabetes, osteoporosis, functional disability, depression and premature death from any cause.

Researchers from the University of Michigan Medicine

used a process of analysis of DNA methylation (also known as age acceleration clocks) to determine biological age and to compare this with grip strength in over 1,200 middle-aged and older adults. Their study found that older biological age correlates closely with weaker grip strength. Muscle weakness was found to be a strong predictor of accelerated and advanced biological ageing measured up to 10 years later.[9]

A grip strength test is quick and easy to perform using a handheld device known as a dynamometer. You simply squeeze the device as hard as possible while seated and with your elbow bent to 90 degrees.

Since the Second World War, Swedish army recruits have undergone a medical examination including grip strength to assess suitability for army duty. This database of young men has been followed up for decades with the finding that, compared to those with moderate or high grip strength, those with lowest grip strength had a 20 per cent increased risk of dying by their mid-50s. Intuitively there is a logic to the importance of grip strength for survival. In times past, being able to carry primitive weaponry, forage for food or climb a tree to escape a predator all utilised grip strength to great effect. Think of Darwin's survival of the fittest becoming survival of the strongest. For older adults, research suggests that rather than following a specific programme of gripping exercises, a wide range of resistance training and forms of other exercise can all support improved grip strength.[10]

Of course, your mindset matters too when it comes to getting stronger. Research from Alia Crum, psychology professor at the Mind and Body Lab at Stanford, has found that your mindset when it comes to health improvement has the capacity to change you physically in and of itself. Which is why I believe in the benefits of consistent action. While the precise amount and type of strength training tailored to specific age groups and individuals remains the subject of ongoing research, there is no doubt that being stronger supports your living better and longer. Personally I have found that setting strength targets and seeing them achieved and then surpassed builds its own motivational momentum in an upward spiral.

If or when going to the gym isn't feasible, don't worry. You can do many strength-based exercises at home using nothing except your own body weight and perhaps some resistance bands to add a further degree of difficulty.

Think about simply standing up and sitting down repeatedly on a chair with a back support, doing step-ups using the bottom step of your stairs or trying modified push-ups against a wall. Everyday household items including cans of beans, bags of oats or watering cans for the gardeners can all provide practical ways to build some strength.

The 'exercise prescription' from lifestyle medicine advocates two or three 20-to-30 minute strength sessions each week, focusing on the main muscle groups. So, what are you waiting for? If you already have a well-established strength-training habit then keep going. If not, then the best time to start is right now, today. Join a gym and start a class. Most of us need support and accountability and simply getting a few classes of instruction can set you up for sustainable progress. A trainer can support you to build that new habit safely and successfully, reducing the risk of injury by helping you to learn the basics of form and function. In fact, simply lifting light weights comfortably at a faster pace can support sustainable improvements in functional capacity and better biological ageing. This is because muscle power is more closely associated with good physical functioning than either the size or strength of the muscles.

The metabolic magic from building more strength means a little less weakness and a little more life. If you don't want to have average strength when you're older, then you need better-than-average habits right now! As you become physically stronger and more agile, you provide your mental and emotional health with an important biological resilience buffer too, while challenging yourself to stay in the zone of peak strength and fitness. The bottom line is that staying strong is about the quality of your everyday life and lived experience. Simply start, today!

Sleep soundly

Restorative sleep is one of the key pillars of lifestyle medicine as it supports your long-term health and wellbeing. Indeed, I often say that your wellbeing today started with the quality of your sleep last night. It really is that important when it comes to mental wellbeing, mood and motivation, in addition to metabolism and optimal brain, heart and immune health. While we know so much more about the science of sleep now compared to several decades ago, it's clear that we are still only scratching the surface in terms of these scientific understandings.

One of the great paradoxes about sleep is that during the period of time when you shut your eyes and rest, as bodily functions slow down your brain becomes or remains very active. There is a significant increase in brain blood flow detected during sleep, while glial cells and the glymphatic system in the brain shrink like a drying sponge as they clear broken bits of DNA and cellular clutter from the brain circuits – essentially clearing out the 'brain trash'.

If you sleep soundly for 7–8 hours a night, remember that you are luckier than the estimated one in every three adults who admit to poor sleep patterns. Many people suffer significant health consequences as a result of short-changing their sleep, including mood swings, memory issues (such as 'brain fog'), high blood pressure, fatigue and weight gain.

Many medical conditions may adversely impact sleep too, including menopause, prostate issues, bladder problems, chronic pain and many others. Caring for a child with behavioural issues can play havoc with sleep patterns, while mental health issues including toxic stress, anxiety and depression often overlap with disturbed sleep. Certain prescription medications can negatively impact sleep, including treatments for heart disease and blood pressure, steroids and antidepressants (SSRIs), over-the-counter decongestants and antibiotics, amongst others.

Very often, poor sleep is symptomatic of a larger under-lying issue that needs to be addressed in terms of either your health or the health of a family member. Taking time to explore and address these can be really important in terms of the health of your future self. Which reminds me of Dave, who had been feeling tired for quite a while by the time he eventually came to see me. Aged 48, he no longer had the energy to go to the gym.

Recent blood tests done as part of a work medical had all returned normal results, while he described no changes to any of his bodily functions. While busy at work as a corporate executive, he hadn't experienced any undue stress either. In fact, since the pandemic, the regular trans-atlantic travel that had been part and parcel of his role was now minimised to a couple of times a year at most.

Was Dave a snorer? I wondered.

'A very loud one,' Dave said. 'It's embarrassing really. It's been going on for a couple of years and my wife, Sinéad, says it's really bad. Her own sleep has been so badly affected by the snoring that she has now been prescribed sleeping tablets by her own doctor.'

Worryingly, Dave had almost nodded off while on a recent long-distance drive, and the occasional Sunday afternoon nap on the couch had become a regular habit for him.

'This was something my grandad used to do when he got older,' said Dave, 'but I never thought it would be something I'd be doing at my age.'

'Do you ever stop breathing during your sleep?' I asked.

'Sinéad says sometimes it's like there's just complete silence for a minute or so,' Dave said. 'She was concerned and convinced me to come see you.'

My thoughts immediately turned to sleep apnoea, an increasingly recognised serious complication of disordered sleep with potentially far-reaching consequences for your health, including increased risks of heart attack, stroke and longer-term memory loss.

An Epworth sleep questionnaire scored Dave in the moderate sleep apnoea category. We arranged for him to have relevant tests done to measure his overnight oxygen saturation levels, which confirmed the diagnosis. Wearing a CPAP mask at night has sorted out his snoring and resolved his apnoea. CPAP (continuous positive airway pressure) keeps the airway open so that you receive the oxygen you need while you sleep. Quite quickly, Dave began to feel much better as his energy improved. He was even finally able to get back to the gym.

His wife, Sinéad, sleeps much better now too, and thankfully has ditched the sleeping tablets. I'm not a fan of them at all, given their risk of tolerance, dependence and addiction. A little-known fact about sleeping tablets is their association with long-term adverse health issues, from an increased risk of falls to increased all-cause mortality.[1] Definitely not something that your future self would thank you for!

Patricia's situation was completely different, as many years of shift work in a local factory had played havoc with her sleep routine. Having availed of a redundancy package a year earlier, she was no longer working irregular hours, but she had been unable to sort out her sleep issues. Her sleep was patchy and broken. At times she would wake up in the middle of the night and be unable to get back to sleep again; other times she couldn't fall asleep at all. Happily married with four grown-up children at 55 years old, she had no major worries or stressors apart from the usual parenting ups and downs. Financially, she was on solid ground with the mortgage paid off and her husband working for the local council in a relatively low-stress job.

When she eventually came to see me about her poor sleep pattern, she felt she was a chronic insomniac. She said she had tried 'everything', so I was keen to explore what 'everything' meant for Patricia. She had seen a hormone specialist (an endocrinologist) who had prescribed hormone replacement therapy a year earlier to treat some of her menopause symptoms. While Patricia felt this had helped her in many aspects of her wellbeing, unfortunately it hadn't improved the quality of her sleep.

Patricia was also aware of the impact of caffeine on sleep quality, limiting her caffeine intake to one cup of coffee each morning. She was careful to avoid caffeine in the second half of the day, choosing chamomile tea instead. A thermostat in her dark bedroom ensured a cooler temperature of about 18 degrees Celsius, and her mattress was comfortable.

The only thing missing from Patricia's list of 'everything' was light – specifically blue light. I explained the science of how early morning exposure to natural blue light (that is, daylight) can set your natural body clock, enhance the body's rhythms and regularise sleep patterns, while late-night exposure to artificial blue light, such as the light from a mobile phone or laptop screen, has the opposite effect – significantly reducing levels of the sleep-inducing hormone melatonin, which signals to both brain and body that darkness and the wind-down for sleep have arrived. Over time Patricia changed her relationship with her mobile phone, no longer taking it to bed and turning it off most evenings by 9 p.m. She also tried to get outdoors to soak in some early morning blue light, which is so beneficial to the circadian rhythm and natural sleep cycle.

While Patricia had indeed tried almost 'everything', she had never gone to a trained therapist about her sleep. The latest recommendation from the European Insomnia Guidelines advocates cognitive behavioural therapy, provided either in person or online, as the first-line treatment for insomnia disorder in adults of any age.[2] On my advice, Patricia went to see an expert that I recommended in this area. Several months later, her sleep has improved significantly and Patricia feels she is reaping the wellbeing benefits on a daily basis.

Awareness of just how fundamental sleep is to how you focus, function and feel every day is a starting point to begin to reprioritise your sleep. Putting sleep near the top of your self-care strategies is such a sound investment in terms of both your everyday lived experience and your future health. As you reduce cellular inflammation, support the immune system and slow down biological ageing, you lower the risks of developing diabetes, depression, dementia, heart disease and stroke.

Benjamin Franklin put it well when writing that 'early to bed and early to rise makes a man healthy, wealthy and wise'. The many everyday benefits of restorative sleep include recharging more fully from stress, feeling more invigorated and having more energy and everyday vitality. A good night's sleep enables you to be more present, focused and attentive. As a foundation stone for willpower, sleep supports healthier food choices, leading to a more balanced metabolism and gut microbiome.

Sleep clears out brain 'clutter' while acting as a catalyst for clarity of thought, creative thinking and consolidation of learning and memory. Think more clearly and feel more revitalised tomorrow while supporting your longer-term health and wellbeing by prioritising your sleep tonight.

Let your lifestyle
be your medicine

Are your everyday lifestyle habits health-enhancing or health-depleting?

Back in 2017, I was honoured to give a TEDx talk in UCD entitled 'The Doctor of the Future: Prescribing Lifestyle as Medicine', which reflects my ongoing advocacy for sustainable health and lasting wellbeing. Thomas Edison once wrote, 'The doctor of the future will give no medicine, but will interest his patient in the care of the human frame, in diet, and in the cause and prevention of disease.' Right now, we are a long way from Edison's predictions. While certainly a noble aspiration, it implies a complete paradigm shift in how we advocate for lasting health and wellbeing, which, of course, is light years from the lived experience and everyday reality for many.

Of course, most disease in the Western world is neither caused by drug deficiency nor cured by those same drugs. Don't get me wrong, modern medicine can be miraculous; think antibiotics for meningitis or pneumonia, clot-busting blood thinners and adrenaline for life-threatening allergic reactions – and then, of course, there are the many surgical interventions that save lives and restore health. Timely medical care can be invaluable if and when you need it.

But for many long-term health conditions, medication can only get you so far. It can help, but doesn't heal the tsunami of chronic, largely lifestyle-related health conditions, from heart disease and high blood pressure to diabetes and dementia. The pill-for-every-ill approach can at best modify or manage them and doesn't have the capacity to reverse or cure them.

The majority of visits to doctors nowadays involve chronic health conditions, which often equate to chronic lifestyle conditions. In other words, these conditions can often be prevented, more successfully managed and potentially even reversed at times through positive lifestyle changes.

Lifestyle as medicine is this new idea (which is actually a very old idea – think Hippocrates' quote about food as medicine) that the small, everyday health and lifestyle choices you make can have a big impact on your healthspan (my term for the number of years you stay healthy) and, with a modicum of good luck, on your lifespan as well. In other words, adding life to your years as well as perhaps years to your life.

That's the essence of the lifestyle medicine message – moving upstream to address the root causes as opposed to simply treating the symptoms. Reinforcing the foundations of sustainable wellbeing as opposed to just putting a sticking plaster on the cracked wall of ill health.

Of course, while you may do everything 'right' in terms of eating healthily, exercising and managing stress well, you may still simply be unlucky and develop a serious illness. That's just a fact. A healthy lifestyle and regular medical check-ups do not guarantee anything, but they do allow you to control the controllables and significantly increase your odds of staying healthy.

One of the most inspirational guests to appear on my wellbeing podcast is Dr Akil Taher, author of a book titled *Open Heart* and a fellow family physician all the way from Alabama, USA. Despite knowing 'what to do' in terms of his own health, he had for years eschewed health habits for a life of chronic overwork and overindulgence in what's referred to as the 'Modern American Diet' (or MAD). From having heart disease and angioplasty at the age of 56 and a near-death cardiac event at the age of 61, his bypass surgery became his tipping point for transformational change. Akil has gone from being a couch potato to climbing Mount Kilimanjaro and running marathons as he continues to challenge himself physically and mentally. He emphasises the important role that food plays in heart and other chronic health conditions as an exponent of a plant-rich, whole-food-based approach to nutrition. He has become an exemplar of the Confucius quote 'We have two lives, and the second begins when we realise we only have one.' As he has healed himself, his message becomes one of hope: it's never too late to take action, to make changes, and simply start to embrace that healthier, more vibrant version of yourself.

The word 'responsibility' is a composite of two separate words – 'response' and 'ability': in other words, your ability to respond in any given situation. This is why responsibility for your own self-care is so important. It's important to appreciate that while there are many things that you cannot control or influence, the one thing you always can do is to make a conscious commitment to take good care of yourself. This is something that many people understandably neglect to do, especially if or when they are busy and stressed or feel overwhelmed. By committing to self-care, you choose to take back ownership of your own wellbeing journey. The many tiny health choices and decisions you make each day add up and compound to move you in a health-enhancing or health-depleting direction. This is where an understanding of the six pillars of lifestyle medicine can be so helpful.

THE SIX PILLARS OF LIFESTYLE MEDICINE
Building positive, supportive relationships
Recharging effectively from stress
Exercise and movement
Restorative sleep
Nutritious food
Avoiding noxious substances

To this, I would add a seventh pillar – spending time in health- and wellbeing-enhancing environments, especially nature and the arts.

The INTERHEART study has found that nine modifiable risk factors could explain more than 90 per cent of the risk of a heart attack, while the majority of strokes can also be prevented.[1] The Diabetes Prevention Program has found that people with pre-diabetes who take part in a structured lifestyle change programme could reduce their risk of developing type 2 diabetes by 58 per cent (71 per cent for people over 60 years old). Overall, about

80 per cent of cases of type 2 diabetes are thought to be preventable.[2]

In terms of mental health, recent research has found that seven separate lifestyle habits (with emphasis on social connection, balanced eating and moderation of alcohol intake) can reduce depression risk by 57 per cent, even where there is a genetic predisposition to depression.

Recently, the *Journal of the American Medical Association* found that a healthy lifestyle positively impacts cognition, as it was associated with a lower dementia risk, even among participants at high genetic risk of developing dementia.[3]

If you imagine your chromosomes as shoelaces, then the protective tips at the end of them represent telomeres, which are made from repeating short sequences of DNA and covered by special proteins. As you age, these telomeres become frayed and don't protect the chromosomes as well, leading to cell malfunction and manifestations of cellular ageing including the onset of chronic disease.

One of the great scientific breakthroughs in recent years has been the discovery of the enzyme telomerase by Dr Elizabeth Blackburn, who received the Nobel Prize in Medicine for her brilliant discovery. She found that telomerase can add DNA to telomeres, which supports their health, protects cells and delays ageing. Not only can this enzyme prevent the telomeres from shortening and slow down ageing, but it may even partially reverse telomere shortening. This research underpins many of the benefits of lifestyle as medicine, as all its pillars have been shown to positively impact telomeres. Exercise and movement are wonderful ways to feel more positive and alive. The concept of food as medicine is gathering momentum as the importance of the microbiome for health becomes better understood. The game-changing benefits of restorative sleep for your mood, memory, motivation and mojo are phenomenal. Recharging from stress and building emotionally rich interpersonal relationships are fundamental for your vitality as a human being. Avoiding noxious substances, including cigarettes, cocaine, and excess alcohol – need I say more?

Research by Dr Dean Ornish published in the prestigious medical journal *The Lancet* has found there to be a dose–response relationship between the degree of lifestyle change and telomerase activity. In other words, the more positive lifestyle change you embrace in terms of the six pillars, the more potent its impact on your telomeres. His research followed men diagnosed with prostate cancer over five years. At the end of the study, those men who had embraced lifestyle changes significantly increased the length of their telomeres over the five-year period, whereas a control group of patients who hadn't embraced lifestyle changes had shorter telomeres.

Of course, there will always be outliers to the healthy-lifestyle-as-medicine message. Whether it's the 85-year-old man who smoked all his life or the 90-year-old woman who never exercised – or, on the flip side, the middle-aged person who took great care of their health and still died early from some non-lifestyle-related fatal condition. Hearing about these stories may make you ask yourself, quite reasonably I may add, 'Why bother changing? Why not just carry on? Sure, I'm grand just the way I am.' And I'm sure you are. But becoming a more active participant in your own wellbeing can have significant long-term benefits. In terms of the hard objective science, you can slash your odds of chronic health conditions and age-linked health problems significantly.

But perhaps even more importantly, a healthy lifestyle can boost your everyday subjective wellbeing. While it can be nice to believe you're going to stay healthier (and maybe even live longer), isn't it even better to feel more energetic and think more clearly? To experience more emotional equanimity and mental clarity, enabling you to think, feel, and be closer to your creative best today, tomorrow, and the day after, while also banking up healthspan benefits well into your twilight years? That's what lifestyle as medicine can offer.

Aged 42 and already a seasoned and successful entrepreneur in the emerging tech space, Michael was 'tuned into' health matters – up to a point. He understood, for example, the importance of managing his asthma and getting early treatment for respiratory infections, which he was prone to. Michael understood the value of proactively managing this condition through taking his inhalers and anti-allergic medication and getting annual flu shots. While his attitude to his asthma care was first class, it wasn't nearly enough to enhance his long-term health and wellbeing.

For years, Michael always seemed to me overly preoccupied with his work – at the expense of everything else in his life. While I tried to encourage him over the years to take more exercise and to spend more time resting and recharging from stress, my words always seemed to fall on deaf ears. I remember seeing Michael one day and being shocked at how the gradual mission creep of his high-octane, stressful and sedentary lifestyle had caught up with him. His belly circumference was up to 45 inches, his sleep was poor as he found it increasingly difficult to 'switch off' at night and he had non-specific aches and pains. While he did admit to having low energy and to making less time than ever for exercise, realigning his life habits simply wasn't on Michael's radar. When I asked how important he thought it was to make some positive lifestyle changes, he rated this at only five out of ten – well below the minimum of seven needed for successful behavioural change.

The next time I saw Michael in my consultation room, about 18 months later, I was very pleased at the evident positive transformation. He looked so much leaner and stronger, and this was backed up by a reduced belly measurement of 39 inches.

It transpired that, shortly after his last visit to me, Michael had been in London for one of his regular conferences. Quite suddenly, while bending to unpack his suitcase in his hotel bedroom, he had developed severe low back pain. It had laid him up for several days, leaving him unable to attend meetings or social events. Michael told me that, for the first time in years, he had quiet time to think, free from distractions, deadlines or any other work-related drama.

'I began to think how my energy had been flagging in recent times,' Michael said. 'I thought about my flabby appearance in the bathroom mirror, about my change in trouser size, about how I couldn't remember the last time I had been able to run up a flight of stairs. And I thought about my favourite uncle, Joe, whose health was ravaged by late-onset type 2 diabetes. And I thought, what good is this career, the status and "success", if I can't feel good and stay healthy?'

Michael jokes that he could hear me in his ear, replaying our last conversation where I had emphasised the importance of staying strong through health-enhancing habits.

Ironically, Michael had always been a strong advocate of my message, having had me speak on burnout prevention and wellbeing on several occasions for his company. But when it came to his own life, he had simply left these ideas at the front door. This was now no longer the case. The 'hotel room incident', as Michael refers to it now, became his tipping point for lasting positive change. Of course, once you know your 'why', the 'how' becomes so much easier. Michael had lacked his 'why', despite having access to bucketloads of knowledge and good advice. Now that he had it, he was slowly making the necessary changes.

Over time and through consistency, Michael developed cast-iron habits using what I term the 'Four M Method' – Movement, Mediterranean, Mindful, Measurement.

Firstly, Movement as medicine. Secondly, a Mediterranean approach to eating habits. Both of these are underpinned by a Mindful practice (whether mindful breathing or meditation) to support awareness and presence – the starting point for learning to make health-enhancing choices. Finally, and perhaps most importantly, Measuring progress through a written journal. Having the self-discipline to regularly review your progress in terms of what actually transpires as opposed to what you planned, in terms of what went well and what didn't (and the reasons why you didn't follow through on your good intentions). This can provide fresh insights into how you can better navigate those situations next time in support of your longer-term goals.

Michael's progress to date has been phenomenal. In his words, 'I haven't needed an antibiotic for my chest in over a year. My energy is so much better. My sleep has improved; I wake now without an alarm clock. To be honest, I haven't felt this good in years. I'm loving the exercise as well, which is key for me – strength classes three times a week, some cardio and lots of walks to keep the head clear.'

Today, Michael is pretty much unrecognisable from his former self, not just in terms of his appearance but in his action-oriented philosophy towards his health going forward. He feels so much better, and his biological markers have improved objectively as well, with fat stores down, cholesterol improved and blood sugar and blood pressure both normal. Having chosen to 'walk the walk' as an active participant in his own wellbeing, he is now reaping the benefits in terms of his health.

You can too! It's all about starting. With the advent of 'lifestyle as medicine', a future of fewer pills-for-every-ill, with more skills and strategies to support positive health, has now arrived in the scientific mainstream. By choosing to integrate small positive habits into your life, you can make things a little bit better, step by step and day by day. That's the lesson that Michael, Dr Akil, and many others have learned through their own experiences. Unlike them, you don't have to wait for those health or heart issues to raise their heads to start.

Your health and wellbeing really are priceless. Simply start today with consistent positive changes to make a big difference, not just to your healthspan but, perhaps more importantly, to your everyday lived experience. The rewards can be immense.

Your Emotional Wellbeing

Daily micromoments of positivity compound over time to create a happier, healthier and more resilient future you.

Count your blessings

Have you spent time today counting your blessings, reflecting on the many aspects of your life for which you can be grateful?

One of the paradoxes about gratitude is that, despite its considerable benefits to wellbeing, it isn't always as easy or natural as it seems. Our brains are hardwired for fear, stress and survival, much like they were thousands of years ago when our ancestors roamed the African savannah. Back then, stopping to appreciate the flowers could have cost you your life, while being constantly alert to danger might have saved you from a sabre-toothed lion. Additionally, the psychological principle of hedonic adaptation – our tendency to always return to our base-line level of happiness no matter what positive or negative life changes may occur – means that we tend to adapt to our material circumstances and take the good things in our lives for granted. I describe this phenomenon as 'Gratitude Deficiency Syndrome'. The underlying cause is a feeling of chronic 'not-enoughness,' triggered by negative comparison with others or the fear of not having – or being – enough. Social media can further fuel feelings of ingratitude, fostering a sense of failure to 'keep up with the Joneses'. With this mindset of scarcity and entitlement, grievances will always outnumber gifts. The pressures and demands of daily life can easily overwhelm any feelings of gratitude we may have.

Paradoxically, when life is challenging or you're struggling, this is when a gratitude practice can benefit you the most. Starting with gratitude means you don't mortgage the wellbeing of your future self for today's stresses.

In my experience, gratitude can be used in at least three distinct ways to enhance your wellbeing and lived experience. I refer to these as grateful awareness, grateful appreciation and grateful allowing.

Grateful awareness is an excellent way to bring more heartfelt gratitude into your life. Spend a few minutes writing about three things you feel grateful for and why. These can be small or significant things, from the past or in the present moment. Writing them down connects your brain to the paper, making this expression of gratitude more intentional and real. My preferred time to practise gratitude is in the early morning when I'm feeling fresh, focused and free from the day's inevitable distractions and busyness. Nighttime, just before sleep, can also be a good time and has the added benefit of promoting a more restorative night's sleep. The key is consistency; as with everything, actions speak louder than words.

When counting your blessings using the 'three good things' exercise, it's essential to be specific and dive deep into details, rather than just making a list. Why do you think that good thing happened? What does it mean to you? Did you share it with anyone? Writing these reflections on paper expands your awareness of the many good things in your life. Don't forget to include life's little things, which can be a source of much happiness and joy – for example, the coffee you enjoyed this morning, a conversation or call from a friend or the comfortable bed you slept in last night.

Grateful appreciation involves taking some time to intentionally acknowledge and appreciate the people in your life right now. Consider how you feel when someone appreciates and thanks you – whether for a small gift, a task completed or an encouraging word. Most people feel valued, validated and glad to receive acknowledgement.

Turning things around, focus on grateful appreciation by consciously choosing to acknowledge, recognise and thank someone else. A simple, meaningful 'thank you' or a kind word of encouragement can make a big difference in someone else's day. Who can you intentionally appreciate today through an active demonstration of gratitude or kindness? Perhaps a friend, family member, work colleague or even the person who makes your cup of coffee?

Finally, the concept of grateful allowing involves non-attachment to setbacks. By non-attachment, I mean not staying stuck in the past, defined by old stories that no longer serve you. Instead, through a process of reframing, you can allow life's inevitable setbacks to become opportunities for growth. One of the interesting aspects of adversity and life's setbacks is that many people eventually describe a deep sense of gratitude for having come through the experience. They develop a renewed appreciation for life and a stronger sense of who they are in the world. Grateful allowing supports a shift in perspective, where you focus on the lessons learned, the strengths you were able to draw upon, how you've grown as a person, and the ways you can now be grateful for the experience – even if you did not feel this way at the time.

This reminds me of Deirdre, who developed a lump in her right breast four years ago. A prompt assessment led to an early invasive cancer diagnosis. While she needed extensive treatment at the time, she recovered well and remains cancer-free to this day. Recently, she described to me how her life had changed since her cancer journey began.

'Being diagnosed with cancer in my early forties was such a shock and a traumatic experience,' Deirdre said. 'It shook me to the core, as I had to confront my mortality for the first time. The chemotherapy was tough, and it took time to recover to the point where I could function somewhat normally again. Alongside this, there was profound fatigue and emotional exhaustion. There were lots of tears too. And yet, looking back on the experience now, I can appreciate how much it has fundamentally changed how I see things. It has given me a deep sense of gratitude and appreciation for having overcome the experience, for being in remission and for the gift of life itself. While I was never an ungrateful person before, I was busy and preoccupied with life's challenges; like many people, I took a lot of things for granted. Looking back now, it's as if I was sleepwalking through life. But when I was at my lowest, gratitude found its way into my heart. Releasing this gratitude has helped me heal and move forward. It has changed my perspective dramatically, becoming the foundation on which I now live my life.'

From a health and wellbeing perspective, cultivating the habit of gratitude can pay rich dividends for your mind, body and soul. Gratitude increases subjective well-being, as you experience more emotional equanimity, and enhances everyday lived experience. It simply isn't possible to feel grateful on the one hand and stressed, anxious or hostile on the other. As a powerful antidote to anxiety and toxic stress, it supports emotional resilience, enabling you to see the world through more grateful eyes as you take stock and appreciate the many gifts your life contains.

Research has found that keeping a gratitude journal just once a week for 10 consecutive weeks can result in participants becoming up to 25 per cent happier, releasing positive emotions that increase your capacity for creativity and joy.[1] Counting your blessings is a terrific way to enhance your emotional bank account with positivity while deepening purpose and a sense of meaning.

Research conducted using fMRI scans has found that gratitude lights up those brain areas that deal with fairness, empathy, motivation, regulation of emotion, stress relief and social support. Expressing gratitude has been associated with enhanced activity in the medial prefrontal cortex, the area linked to learning and decision-making. The effect of gratitude on the brain may last for a long time, too, making the brain more sensitive to gratitude as time passes, meaning that gratitude as a practice can lead to an ever more 'grateful brain.'[2]

One of the key takeaways is that you don't need to do this gratitude exercise every day. Counting your blessings once or twice a week is enough to reap the wellbeing benefits while keeping the exercise fresh and interesting.

Physically, gratitude can move you away from a stressed, high-cortisol state of concern towards its polar opposite – the restorative relaxation response. This occurs when the body's parasympathetic nervous system is activated, also known as the 'pause and plan' or 'rest and digest' state. This is perhaps why gratitude is associated with better sleep, a stronger immune system, and even a lowering of blood pressure.[3] Regularly practising gratitude for as few as six weeks can enhance mental wellbeing and boost resilience while reframing your perspective on life through a more grateful lens. As a result of being grateful, you are more likely to value and take better care of yourself, supporting the health of current and future you.[4]

Several years ago, I gave a keynote talk in London to a number of tech entrepreneurs. They were high achievers, and they were all highly stressed and living on the edge. My wellbeing message resonated with many of these techies who were grappling with the double-edged sword of stratospheric success and serious (and in some cases, majorly debilitating) stress. However, a comment made near the end of the talk by one attendee has always stayed with me.

'All this talk of gratitude is complete nonsense,' he said. 'I mean, we are never going to drive on and build a billion-dollar company if we spend our time feeling grateful. We need to be hungry to have success.'

I thanked him for his very insightful comment and explained one of the important myths about gratitude – that it turns ambition or drive into a damp squib of self-satisfied smugness. Far from it. In fact, gratitude generates enormous forward momentum from a place of abundance and appreciation.

Research that got participants to set several personal goals over a period of 10 weeks looked at the impact of a weekly written gratitude practice. It found that those in the 'gratitude group' made 20 per cent more progress towards their goals and worked harder on those goals both during the 10 weeks and afterwards in the longer term. Their gratitude practice acted like a glue, strengthening and supporting their desire to achieve their goals. Regularly counting their blessings built grit and persistence, fuelling further progress towards those goals.

THE HEALTH BENEFITS OF GRATITUDE

- Reduces stress and anxiety
- Strengthens immune system
- Reduces depressive feelings

- Boosts inner happiness by up to 25 per cent
- Increases capacity for creativity
- Increases empathy
- Improves sleep
- Enhances mental and physical health
- Improves psychological adaptation to major life changes or health challenges
- Builds resilience to life's stressors
- Fuels progress towards personal goals
- Provides the 'glue' to support new habits
- Supports spiritual wellbeing

When you count your blessings, you become less stressed and more peaceful, less reactive and more responsive, less resistant and more accepting of change. Gratitude can bring hope in the face of despair, light in the face of darkness and healing in the face of brokenness. Overall, people who are grateful tend to be healthier and happier, more empathic and helpful, more forgiving, more spiritual, less materialistic and simply more likeable. What might you be blind to in your life right now that you could see more clearly through the lens of gratitude and appreciation? Count your blessings and practise gratitude to build a solid foundation to your life – strengthening your relationships, supporting your physical health, and improving your wellbeing while opening up a heart that is a rich reservoir of positivity.

Reframe the hurt

Think for a moment about something in your own life that has given you a great sense of personal satisfaction – something that has made you feel really proud. Perhaps it's an academic achievement or a professional accomplishment, a challenge you overcame, an award you won or simply a very small personal 'win' that meant a lot to you.

For me, the proud moment that comes to mind is when I first started my own medical practice. It was the beginning of a whole new adventure for me. I was renting a space over a corner shop in a housing estate, right across the road from where I had grown up and where my parents still lived at the time, so it was very local and very personal. From day one, I had thrown myself with gusto into the challenge and worked hard to provide a warm and welcoming space for our growing community of patients. While it was incredibly exciting, it was daunting on another level: grappling with the responsibility of becoming an employer, arranging a bank overdraft, purchasing practice equipment and all that goes with starting a small business. Not for the faint hearted.

We took great pride in the little things that made our space uniquely special and homely, like the fresh blue paint on the walls and the comfortable waiting area. There were leather chairs from our own home, while some prints that we had received as wedding gifts adorned the walls. We even had our own coffee machine back then, which was quite something in pre-Celtic Tiger Ireland!

Time passed by, and everything was ticking along nicely. Until one fateful day almost a year after the practice opened. It was the early morning of Friday 25 February when there was knock on my front door – impatient, loud and hurried. I rushed downstairs in my pyjamas and opened it to see a Guard standing there. He asked if I was the doctor, Mark Rowe, and I nodded.

'You'd better come quickly,' he said. 'Your medical practice is on fire.'

It was as if time stood still. I recall getting dressed and driving the 10 minutes to the surgery, my mind racing.

How could this happen? Was there an electrical fault? Had the fire started in the local convenience store downstairs? What damage had been done?

When I arrived, my worst fears were realised. The damage was immense and the premises was ruined. The emergency services had been exemplary; the fire brigade had already done their job in extinguishing the flames, though smoke was still billowing from the upstairs windows. Several of the neighbours had gathered around, watching the unfolding inferno. Some had the morning newspaper and fresh 'blaas' (bread rolls, a Waterford delicacy) in hand; a reminder that, as always, life goes on. My life-changing 'event' was simply of momentary interest to others as part of their morning routine, and a footnote perhaps in the day's events for others. For me though, at that moment, it was all consuming. All I could see was my livelihood, my future, everything I had worked so hard for literally going up in smoke in front of my eyes. I felt numb.

After a couple of hours had passed by, it was deemed safe enough to enter the premises. I'll never forget the smell that hit me as I climbed the soot-stained steps of the stairs – a powerful, pungent stench of smoke and charred wood. If you've ever experienced a fire you'll know immediately what I'm talking about.

As I reached the top of the stairs, my attention was drawn to what looked like the remains of a red party balloon stuck to the corner of the wall. Getting closer, I realised it was what remained of the fire extinguisher. The computers and coffee machine were melted beyond recognition. The once-cheerful waiting area, with its bright blue walls and carefully chosen prints, now more closely resembled a dark, dank cave. This memory of how black everything appeared covered by charcoal dust has stayed with me to this day.

As I surveyed the scene it seemed surreal, like a bad dream. Of course, your fight-or-flight response kicks into overdrive and survival instincts take over. We were doctors and had people who depended on us. To add to the sense of surrealness, there was even a lady sitting in a parked car outside the premises looking for (and eventually receiving) an anti-inflammatory painkilling injection for back pain.

For our small team of five people – my medical colleague, nurse and two administrators – the situation was stark, but the show had to go on. We sat down as a team to figure out a way forward, drew up a long 'to do' list and got to it. We worked throughout the weekend to open again in a temporary premises across the road – not the homely place we had created a year earlier, but it was functional. We were sending a message to the world that we would carry on no matter what. That we were bulletproof.

However, behind the veneer of bravado and invincibility, the 'show' didn't go on quite as smoothly for me – partly because this incident had happened on my own doorstep, but mainly because it represented my dreams being crushed. Deliberately. Footage from CCTV cameras showed two hooded youths entering our upstairs premises, bypassing the side entrance to the shop downstairs, which remained untouched. Analysis at the scene revealed that several separate fires had been set. Far from being an electrical fault or freak accident, this was deliberate arson.

Who was despicable enough to do such a thing? Why did they do it? Would they – whoever 'they' were – come to my home next? These thoughts consumed me. My sense of safety and security in the world was badly shaken.

Although some of our patients came forward to say that they knew who set the fire, and the police charged somebody eventually, the resultant trial collapsed and ended in a mistrial. To this day, it remains an unsolved case.

Looking back now, it was a fraught and hectic time. I was working around the clock. Days and weeks passed by in a haze and I was on constant high alert. Toxic stress can have a very corrosive impact on your wellbeing, and I was no exception. Without many of the 'staying well' practices that are second nature to me nowadays, I struggled. I had difficulty sleeping and frequent nightmares and I was constantly on edge, ruminating and recycling negative thoughts repeatedly. Worse still were my feelings of guilt for having 'poor me syndrome'; after all, nobody got burned or hurt in the fire and as a doctor I meet people who deal so bravely with far worse things in the form of illnesses and health challenges every single day.

After a few weeks of being consumed by thoughts of the arson attack, I did what I would advise many of my patients to do and went to speak to someone about it. Talk therapy, sometimes known as cognitive behavioural therapy or CBT, is based on the idea that by examining your thoughts and your beliefs about those thoughts, you can learn to see things differently. It can be an extremely effective way to support you in navigating all sorts of life challenges and is something everyone can potentially benefit from at different times. I was no exception. Just one session provided the cathartic release I needed.

One of the best lessons I've ever learned is that while I couldn't change what had happened, I could choose how to respond. I had to choose to see things differently, to let go of the fire and the need to know 'why', and instead to embrace the gift of acceptance. To accept what had happened and to move on.

That arson attack taught me so much about resilience. We all face metaphorical fires in our lives. Oftentimes these fires are external – challenging life events that impact our health or relationships or finances. But while experiencing pain is one of the great inevitabilities of life, the setbacks and struggles we face can lead to growth and new perspectives. Every experience can provide the opportunity to learn and to grow, developing a better sense of your strengths and who you are, with a deeper sense of meaning and appreciation for life itself. There's no doubt in my mind that the fire changed the trajectory of my life. Less than 18 months later, I had built a brand-new, 4000-square-foot facility and taken on more support staff. The practice grew rapidly and subsequently moved again to the Waterford Health Park, where it has been located for the last 15 years.

Sometimes synchronicities pop up in our field of awareness. If we are open and pay attention, they can provide us with new insights. So it was with a long-standing patient of mine, Derek. He had spent many years working in construction as a block-layer and during the boom times the money was flowing. Often quite literally, as Derek's dependence on alcohol began to take hold. Eventually he realised that this habit was beginning to destroy all that was good in his life. With my support, he was accepted into a treatment programme and did well. Regularly attending aftercare, Derek was well on the road to recovery with a new job and brighter future on the horizon.

Two years passed and one Monday morning Derek attended the practice, panicky, agitated and highly anxious. He was teary eyed as he disclosed that he had been bingeing on cocaine for some time, and recently it had, in his own words, 'got out of hand'.

That weekend, in a fit of coke-induced rage and paranoia, he had set fire to a warehouse he had recently been employed as a security guard to protect. This had all been captured on CCTV footage, with Derek readily identifiable. He had already been arrested and serious charges were now pending.

Here was a real-life version of the nameless, faceless arsonist I had 'encountered' more than 20 years earlier. But instead of the hooded menace that once haunted my nightmares, it was a vulnerable man I knew well. I liked Derek and I had always admired him for his commitment to recovery. No matter my personal feelings about what he had done, Derek had come to me seeking help. With my continued support, he went back to treatment for three months with a great outcome.

I've never met a strong person with an easy past, a successful person who didn't at one point in time fail or a wise person who hasn't made naive mistakes. Derek now leads his recovery support group while actively pursuing a career as an addiction counsellor. Reflecting on Derek's story, I now know deep down that my experience of the arson attack many years earlier had been a great teacher. Learning to accept what had happened and move on built tenacity and grit, while the immediate aftermath gave me a valuable lesson in sustainable self-care. It was an important part of my own journey, showing me how to see things differently and how to move the conversation from 'what I have lost' to 'how I can grow'. And that's my hope for you too. That you face the outer fires in your own life with courage, conviction and self-compassion. That they become sparks of opportunity to grow and to become wiser, stronger and better.

But there is also an inner fire that exists within each and every one of us. Your inner fire keeps you vibrant, just as your pulse and body temperature keep you alive. The essence of stoking your inner fire is saying 'yes' to life and all that is good in your life today. Yes to awareness, to abundance and to gratitude. Yes to health, to friendships and to nature. Yes to all that makes you come alive through how you express yourself. Yes to having the courage to seek support, to choose closure and healing. Yes to finding the light instead of staying stuck in darkness. Yes to reframing your hurts so you can shine more brightly in the world. Yes to future you!

Give back and help others

The Greek philosopher Aristotle once surmised that the essence of life is 'to serve others and do good'. There has never been a greater need for philanthropy in the world and there are so many ways to give back and help others, from donating to charities doing work globally, to supporting the work of researchers that will impact humanity, to helping out with local community efforts. Living your values, being an example to others and giving social support are all ways that you can make the world that little bit more decent, dignified and interdependent.

The ubiquitous 'golden rule' which has existed in almost all cultures and civilisations for centuries tells us to 'treat others as you would like to be treated'. Generosity and kindness are the embodiment of this golden rule. Generosity may be defined as 'giving good things to others freely and abundantly'.[1] Kindness is a character strength for many people as well as a wellbeing practice that can be cultivated and developed. After all, seeking to find the best in others tends to bring out the best in yourself.

From a very early age, we seem to derive wellbeing benefits from giving. One interesting study found that two-year-old toddlers displayed more happiness when giving treats to a puppet rather than themselves, especially when those treats came from the child's own bowl.[2]

The 'giving brain' is a hardwired tendency to give, share and support others as human beings, and has a strong neurobiological basis. Giving to others creates extra brain activity in areas linked to the processing of pleasure and reward (the ventral striatum) influenced by dopamine, and the empathic, trusting, caring part (supra-marginal gyrus of the prefrontal cortex) influenced by oxytocin. In one study, fMRI brain scans were used to record neural activity in participants who were asked to decide how to split 100 dollars between themselves and a local food bank. Activation of the ventral striatum was seen in donors to the food bank, suggesting that giving really is its own reward.[3]

Back in the 1970s, research examining the potential impact of high-fat diets on heart health was carried out using genetically identical New Zealand white male rabbits. This was at a time when the association between a diet high in saturated fat and heart disease was still under investigation. The rabbits were continuously fed the equivalent of a 'heart attack on a plate', a high-saturated-fat diet, for months on end. Not surprisingly, all had similarly high cholesterol levels at the end of the study. Analysis of the lining of their blood vessels, however, revealed that one group of rabbits had 60 per cent fewer fatty deposits in their coronary arteries. This was perplexing. How could genetically identical rabbits, fed the same food in the same environment, have such different outcomes?

Initially, the researchers thought there was a problem with the study. But then they discovered that the heart-healthier rabbits had been cared for by Murina Levesque. Described as a particularly caring and kind individual, Murina had handled the rabbits under her care differently; picking them up, petting them and talking gently to them while nurturing them with kindness and love. It was an intriguing, if inexplicable, association, so they repeated the research under strict conditions. Once more, they found the same results, with similar heart-protective benefits resulting from experiencing kindness: the rabbits cared for by Murina remained healthy, while the others developed severe heart disease. These results were published in the journal *Science* and, like much good research, remained largely ignored until 'rediscovered' by Dr Kelli Harding and described in her 2019 book *The Rabbit Effect: Live Longer, Happier, and Healthier with the Groundbreaking Science of Kindness*. It creates a compelling case for the wellbeing benefits of kindness; perhaps being the recipient of real kindness, care and love is the natural antidote to the stress of modern life that we can all benefit from.[4]

As the rabbit study shows, kindness supports and enhances the wellbeing of recipients of kindness. Furthermore, it brings a plethora of wellbeing benefits to the giver. Witnessing or recalling an act of kindness, or 'prosocial behaviour', also brings forth these very same benefits, meaning that kindness potentially has a three-fold impact on the giver, recipient and observer (whether observed in person or online). It can make you three times as likely to pay the kindness forward in the following 24 hours. Furthermore, kindness is contagious too, spreading several degrees of separation through your community and network.

Giving builds human connection, acting like a glue to strengthen and support relationships. It improves your relationship with yourself too, as you see yourself through a more positive lens, supporting self-esteem and self-worth.

Giving and being generous to others may be one of the best anti-anxiety strategies of all, acting as a circuit breaker on stress, reducing psychological problems, building resilience and boosting wellbeing. Serotonin, oxytocin and dopamine are all increased, supporting your mood and paying into your 'emotional bank account'. Giving supports a more open mind, keeping you other-centred rather than introspective and self-obsessed. Being oriented to consider and care for others builds connection and a resilience buffer to better cope with life's challenges.[5]

Giving supports better mental health – as long as the giver doesn't feel overwhelmed by the demands on his or her time, energy and resources, which may be associated with a worsening of mental wellbeing. As with everything, it's a balancing act – giving to others but not at the expense of giving to yourself in terms of your sustainable self-care needs.

For optimal psychological wellbeing, self-determination theory posits that we have three separate needs that must be met. These are relatedness, competence and autonomy. Giving to others in a way that supports these three separate aspects of self-determination maximises the wellbeing benefits of giving. Relatedness is social connection – developing or deepening a relationship through giving or spending time with the recipient. Competence implies having an understanding of how the giving will be used to impact a recipient or charity, and autonomy means that, as the giver, you have the freedom to choose precisely what you give.[6]

A study was carried out involving participants who were approached in public places and asked to report their subjective happiness level. They were then randomly assigned to four separate groups, being given either five or twenty dollars to spend on themselves or on others. When contacted that evening, those who had been asked to spend their money on others were happier than those who spent personally on themselves, irrespective of the amount. The bottom line was that, in terms of happiness, how you spent your money (on others rather than on yourself) was more important than how much money you had been given. Even five dollars spent on others was enough to increase subjective levels of happiness.[7]

There are so many ways to practise kindness and appreciation that plug into values such as compassion, empathy and gratitude. From volunteering to small acts of kindness such as holding a door or buying someone a coffee, sharing a smile, donating to a worthy cause or helping others, the art of kindness is simple: giving generously and unconditionally.[8]

Over a six-week period, participants were asked to perform random acts of kindness. Those who were instructed to do these kind acts for themselves had no reported emotional benefits afterwards. However, doing five random acts of kindness for others on a single day of the week led to a reported increase in positive emotions and a reduction in negative emotions.

When you do five random acts of kindness on one single day of the week, it makes you more attuned to your thoughts, feelings and actions on that day; makes you more aware of being in the moment in terms of your time; and makes you more appreciative of the impact that your words or actions are having, not only on other people, but on yourself. Interestingly, performing these random acts of kindness over the entire week doesn't seem to work nearly as well, as their positive impact tends to be overshadowed and diluted by everything else going on in your life.

Volunteering can be a natural antidote to negativity and provide an engaging escape from the day-to-day routine. While encouraging a more positive view on life, giving to others through volunteering can allow you to develop new skills or interests, avail of new experiences, become a more rounded and balanced person and help fulfil several important psychological needs, including the need to feel valued. A meta-analysis of 37 observational studies found that, having controlled for factors including financial and health status, 70 per cent of older volunteers reported a greater quality of life than non-volunteers.[9]

Volunteering can improve mood, lower anxiety and reduce the risk of depressive symptoms. By committing to a shared activity, you get to meet people with common interests. Strengthening this sense of interdependence and connection is a strong factor in increasing happiness and wellbeing. Being 'other-centred' can also bring on a helper's high: initial positive emotion followed by more prolonged feelings of emotional contentment. Even simply thinking about donating money or helping others can release these feel-good brain chemicals.

Physical health is also supported by actively volunteering as it lowers stress hormone levels. Perhaps volunteering is a good way to increase physical activity among older adults, which in turn improves physical health. Perhaps those who volunteer are healthier to begin with. Perhaps providing practical help to others offers some protection from the impact of stress on mortality, leading to lower blood pressure and lower all-cause mortality.[10]

A study of volunteering among over 1,200 Americans over the age of 65 found that any amount of volunteering for just one organisation and for less than 40 hours a week led to delayed death. Further research among older Californians found a more than 60 per cent reduced likelihood of dying during the five-year study period compared to those who hadn't volunteered.[11]

Volunteering can also strengthen relationships within organisations, creating a shared common purpose, building positivity and enhancing job satisfaction. As you feel more socially connected, your giving creates a protective buffer against loneliness and depression. By regularly volunteering, you can improve the wellbeing of your community while living better (and perhaps longer) yourself. A real win-win.

Most people, deep down, want to make a meaningful contribution to their community and to be part of something bigger than themselves. Giving back to others supports purpose and meaning, which further enhances long-term health, wellbeing and connection. Mother Teresa put it so well when she said, 'Not all of us can do great things. But we can do small things with great love.'

That idea resonated with me recently as I reflected on an essay called 'The Star Thrower', also known as 'the starfish story', written in 1969 by Loren Eiseley. The story goes like this: an old man was in the habit of walking on the beach each morning before he began his work as a writer. One day, after a big storm had passed, the beach was littered with starfish as far as the eye could see. As the man walked the beach, he noticed a small boy approaching. Every so often, the boy stopped to bend down, pick a starfish up, and throw it into the sea. As the boy drew close, the man asked what he was doing. The boy answered that he was throwing the starfish back into the sea so they wouldn't die later that day when the sun grew strong. The man replied that there were thousands of the starfish on the beach, and the little boy's actions weren't going to make much of a difference.

With that, the boy bent down and picked up a starfish from the glistening sand. Turning toward the ocean, he threw it with all his might. As the starfish disappeared without a trace into the sky-blue water, he turned towards the man and, smiling, said, 'It made a difference to that one.'

Being a giver may change how you see the world, emphasising cooperation over competition, interdependence over independence and togetherness over self-absorption. Mutually supportive relationships require generosity and giving to flourish. Sometimes, giving your time is all that's needed; sometimes, simply giving someone the benefit of the doubt. There are so many worthy organisations out there waiting for you to lend them a hand, so what are you waiting for? Get into the wellbeing habit of generous giving for its own sake, no matter how small the gift or gesture. Small acts of generosity can have a big impact.

Stress less

The plains of the Serengeti in East Africa may seem an unlikely location for cutting-edge research on stress, yet this is exactly where one of the world's leading experts on the stress response, Stanford researcher and neurobiologist Robert Sapolsky, chose to spend time studying the impact of stress on zebras.

In his book *Why Zebras Don't Get Ulcers*, Sapolsky describes how the stress response is primed to keep you alive. A quick burst of speed for a few minutes allows the zebra to escape the chasing lion. Assuming the zebra survives, there is no subsequent postmortem – the zebra doesn't ponder what happened or worry about what might happen next. It simply switches off its stress response and returns to leisurely grazing on the plains of the Serengeti.[1]

If only life's stressors could be switched on and off so easily for us as humans. One of the great attributes of the human brain is its capacity for independent thought. This executive brain function enables you to figure things out and find ways to survive and thrive, all while fine-tuning your interactions with the world day in and day out. Of course, a downside of thinking is too much thinking. Research suggests you may have more than 6,000 predominantly negative thoughts a day. Too many thoughts about the past can trigger resentment and regret, while too many future-oriented thoughts can foster fear, anxiety, worry and insecurity. Because of the negativity bias of your brain, primed for fear detection and survival, you may experience anticipatory stress, worrying about many things – most of which never happen.

This reminds me of Judith, a self-admitted 'born worrier'. She worried about everything and had done all her life. With a pessimistic mindset, she constantly ruminated and recycled negative thoughts and concerns. For years, she was able to keep this pattern of thinking under control – just about. But then a bad breakup and a significant role change in her workplace tipped her over the edge. By the time she came to see me, she had been sleeping poorly, waking several times a night. She felt increasingly stressed and anxious and had experienced a couple of panic attacks. Like many people dealing with toxic stress, she had withdrawn even further into herself and stopped exercising. Her caffeine intake had skyrocketed, and she had become quite fond of a regular glass of wine – or three.

At my suggestion, Judith sought counselling in the form of cognitive behavioural therapy to help her manage her significant anxiety. The talk therapy helped her learn to quiet her inner chatter, dispute negative thoughts and see things differently. By keeping a written journal, Judith became more attuned to her thinking patterns and better able to reframe events in a more positive light. While simply writing things down as a self-help strategy might sound too good to be true, it can and does work. It's well recognised that journalling can buffer stress, build resilience and enhance long-term wellbeing.

In tandem, Judith also benefited from making significant positive lifestyle changes. Learning to prioritise her sleep meant implementing a proper, technology-free wind-down period for at least 90 minutes before bed. Cutting out alcohol completely for three months also greatly improved her wellbeing. Judith hadn't realised how even relatively small amounts of alcohol could negatively impact sleep quality while increasing feelings of anxiety and stress the next day. She reduced her caffeine intake to her non-negotiable one or two cups in the morning, but cut out afternoon caffeine once she understood its negative impact on the 'sleep switch'.

Judith began to focus more on the simple things in her days that provided pleasure, purpose and meaning – like exercise, fresh air, friendships and self-care. She also found solace in connecting with nature and cultivating stillness, helping her shift from her head to her heart. Step by step, she embraced her stress symptoms through sustainable self-care strategies, allowing Judith version 2.0 to emerge, stronger and more at ease with herself and life overall.

Judith's story of suffering from toxic stress is all too common nowadays. Research published in *American Psychologist* highlights that over the past 20 years, people report experiencing stressful events more frequently and feeling more stressed by them. This includes work pressures, deadlines, financial concerns, illness, and both physical health issues and mental health challenges, such as low self-esteem, anxiety, and depression.[2] Add in the turmoil of addiction, loneliness or isolation, and it's easy to understand why many people are experiencing symptoms of toxic stress. There is, quite literally, so much to worry about – from global warming to geopolitical conflicts, not to mention the impact of both mainstream and social media, with endless stories of danger and fear keeping you on high alert. There's never been so much to stress over.

Let's take a closer look at the potential impact of toxic stress on the brain. From impacting the growth of new brain cells to altering brain structure, chronic stress can be harmful and corrosive to the brain in many ways. As an energy-intensive organ, your brain consumes more than 20 per cent of the body's energy, despite making up only 2 per cent of your body weight. Stress burns brain energy rapidly, leading to cravings for comfort foods as depleted brain cells demand more sugar and fuel.

The 'merry-go-mind' of racing, anxious and negative thoughts can diminish your capacity for creativity and innovative thinking. This can overstimulate the amygdala – the brain's 'red button' for reactivity to stress – and weaken its connections to the hippocampus, or memory centre. As a result, you may lose a sense of perspective and context. This can literally change how you think and perceive things, with the brain prioritising short-term reactivity over long-term perspective and responsiveness.

Areas of the brain known as the insula and striatum can become highly activated by chronic stress, leading to feelings of being stuck in a rut and ruminative thoughts of panic, inadequacy, disconnection, despair and emptiness. These negative emotions are difficult to simply 'shake off', and your mood may spiral downward, dampening your ability to cultivate positive emotions. Overall, this can have a negative impact on motivation, performance, productivity and relationships.

But chronic stress doesn't just impact the brain; it can also have significant adverse physical consequences, as it may deplete your energy, leaving you feeling flat and fatigued. Chronic stress can impact the immune system, both directly through the corrosive effects of stress hormones and indirectly by influencing poorer health choices.[3]

Stress hormones such as cortisol increase under conditions of chronic stress. The resultant spike in insulin levels promotes visceral fat storage, which can trigger insulin resistance and other conditions associated with chronic inflammation – including high blood pressure, heart disease, obesity, diabetes, depression and dementia. As chronic stress seeps into your cells, cellular inflammation can damage your telomeres, the protective tips of your chromosomes. Shortened telomeres can impair the mitochondria, the 'batteries' of the cells, causing them to age prematurely and enter a state of irreversible decline. Over time, these damaged cells are unable to divide or stay healthy and eventually die off.

Research by psychologist Janice Kiecolt-Glaser has shed light on how stress can affect metabolism. Her work found two fascinating things; firstly, experiencing social stress within an hour of eating can result in the metabolic equivalent of consuming over a hundred extra calories. This translates to more than 11 extra pounds a year (based on 365 days, 104 extra calories per day, and 3,500 calories per pound). Secondly, stress can alter how certain foods are metabolised. The takeaway? A more mindful approach to eating and properly unwinding from daily stress before meals can benefit your weight, waistline and long-term wellbeing.

Imagine living in a world without stress: no busyness, no noise, no pressure. Sounds perfect, right? Maybe, but it's also pure fantasy. Stress is an integral part of even the most rewarding and fulfilling aspects of life – raising children, achieving career success or pursuing passions. You can't eliminate or eradicate all sources of stress in life, nor should you wish to. The stress response is a key survival tool that helps you respond to challenges and potential threats, whether real or perceived. It's something that, ideally, helps rather than hinders your performance. Experiencing brief periods of stress followed by recovery can actually benefit you in many ways, helping build resilience and allowing you (and your cells) to stay sharper, more agile and biologically younger. Positive anxiety, such as the kind you may feel before an important event, is your body preparing to support enhanced levels of performance, confidence and growth.

Of course, prolonged toxic stress can corrode your wellbeing, which is why it's essential to recharge from stress whenever possible. This starts with being aware of the level of stress you're under, recognising your stress triggers and understanding the potential impact stress is having on your health and wellbeing.

Imagine a traffic light with three colours: red, orange and green. Red represents real threat and danger, where your fight-or-flight response kicks in to avert harm and escape a dangerous situation. Think of the zebra on the Serengeti. Short-lived acute stress followed by recovery is not only a key survival tool but can actually be beneficial; the problems arise when the light stays red for too long, leading to potential harm.

Orange represents the reality many people face daily. While neither life-threatening nor acute, feelings of smouldering low-grade stress permeate everyday living. Think of the many competing demands on your time and energy: work deadlines, distraction from digital devices, financial pressures and the many challenges that life brings. Feelings of loneliness, isolation or disconnection can exacerbate this stress, compounded by poor lifestyle habits like consuming ultra-processed foods or alcohol, overusing social media and not getting enough quality sleep.

Ironically, while you may be acutely aware of what's happening in the outer world, you might be unaware of how this stress is affecting your inner world. Imagine the sound of a fire alarm going off where you are right now. Would you sit there all day with the alarm blaring? Of course not! If it was a real fire, you'd get up and head for the exit. If it was a false alarm, you'd reset it. But in contrast, the inner alarm in your amygdala can stay active all day long, triggered by various stressors. Ignoring it can have significant negative impacts on your wellbeing. Many people spend their time in this orange zone, while reacting internally as if they were in the red zone. The result? Your cells are essentially marinating in cortisol.

Further research by Sapolsky found that if you can't distinguish between an immediate, 'red' stressor and something non-threatening in the orange zone, you'll experience twice the level of stress hormones. This is why it's important to tune in when you're under stress and respond by turning down the stress response and building in regular circuit breakers to recharge.

This brings us to green – the recharge zone, where you return to your true nature by activating the parasympathetic nervous system. You might do this by using self-care strategies, spending time in nature or engaging in activities that bring joy or a state of flow. Being in the green zone may mean pursuing hobbies, joining group classes or just having dedicated time for light-heartedness and laughter.

Other activities in the green zone might include deep relaxation exercises, yoga, tai chi, qi gong, prayer, rhythmic breathing and mindfulness meditation, where your body experiences low psychological and physiological arousal. Everyone can benefit from more time in this green zone for deep rest and restorative recharge.

The key to managing stress optimally is to fine-tune your traffic light response system. Awareness of the zone you're in at any given moment helps you make informed choices to support a transition to a healthier state. You are hardwired to detect danger and trigger the fight-or-flight response, but you are also designed to disconnect from the demand-led stresses of everyday life and reconnect with your true self. I'm a big fan of Epictetus, the Stoic philosopher who emphasised the importance of distinguishing between the many things you can't control, or what I call your circle of concern, and the few things you can, what I call your circle of control. By focusing more energy on what you can control – mainly your own attitude and daily choices – you expand your circle of control and make your circle of concern smaller and less significant.

By attuning your awareness to this traffic light system, you can reduce the hold that toxic stress has on you and learn to let go. It doesn't mean people or situations will stop pushing your buttons or that you'll never overreact. But this new insight into your stress response, and your ability to react appropriately, gives you a path to inner freedom. You become better able to accept uncertainty and embrace change with attentive awareness in the present moment. You become more patient, understanding that many of life's so-called problems resolve themselves; more pragmatic, accepting the things you can't change while finding the courage to change what you can; and more persistent, valuing progress over perfection. You start seeing the bigger picture with a renewed sense of perspective. You become more compassionate toward yourself and others. Ultimately, you become more present, enabling you to fully embrace life as it unfolds – one step, one breath, and one day at a time.

Make time for awe

In 2017 I travelled to Sedona, Arizona, for professional certification in the emerging field of lifestyle medicine. The rugged landscape reminded me of the old cowboy movies from my childhood. After the exam, a group of us spontaneously decided to visit the Grand Canyon. As the bus approached the edge, I was filled with a sense of transcendence. The sheer vastness of the view and the breathtaking panorama before me were almost beyond description. I felt goosebumps rise on my skin, utterly mesmerised by the intensity of the experience. It was a profound sense of connection to something much larger than myself. This was awe.

In the *Oxford English Dictionary*, awe is defined as 'a feeling of reverential respect mixed with fear or wonder'. Many of us experience awe as a transcendent moment of wonder or amazement in the presence of nature, inspiring art, architecture or a spiritual or sporting event.

Standing inside La Sagrada Familia in Barcelona, marvelling at the vibrant stained-glass and rainbow-like reflections inside the grand cathedral – this was awe. Exploring Inisheer, with its ancient stone forts and meandering walls that have stood for thousands of years – this was awe.

Closer to home, there are countless everyday opportunities to experience awe, just waiting for your attention. Awe isn't limited to once-in-a-lifetime moments; it can be found in everyday experiences. Whether it's the early morning dew, a magical sunrise, birdsong, a radiant sunset, windswept sand dunes or the simple smile of a baby, awe can be found wherever you choose to look. Allowing yourself the space to nurture daily micromoments of awe is a powerful way to reconnect with the world in a positive way while enhancing your wellbeing.

Experiencing awe leads to wonder and a psychological state of mystery akin to a childlike curiosity. Awe encourages an openness to new ideas and possibilities, engaging your senses to fully respond to and savour the sounds, scents, scenes and sensations around you. In doing so, it deepens your relationship with the world.

THE AWESOME BENEFITS OF AWE

A: Antidote to stress

W: Wonder and inspiration

E: Enhances health (supports immune function and lowers inflammation)

S: Satisfaction with life increases

O: Other-centred, in terms of connectedness, cooperation and kindness

M: More curious and creative

E: Emotional wellbeing and happiness increase

Imagine taking a weekly walk in an inspiring environment, ideally in nature, perhaps near water or in a wooded garden. Perhaps you go to witness a sunrise or sunset, or to admire architectural beauty in a city. During this walk, you take selfies and report on how you feel – whether stressed, anxious, depressed or happy. This was the essence of the 'awe walk', a study developed with neuroscientist Virginia Sturm.[1] A sample group of 'awe walkers' were compared to a control group who took a fast weekly walk, without focusing on awe.

Three significant findings emerged in the 'awe walking' group. First, as the weeks went by, those exposed to awe experienced an upward spiral, noticing an increase in awe-inspiring moments over time. While people generally tend to adapt to their environment or circumstances over time, gradually returning to their baseline level of happiness (a principle called hedonic adaptation), this didn't happen with the awe-enhancing experiences reported by this group. Second, participants in the awe group demonstrated the 'small self' effect, where the selfies they took showed less and less of themselves and more of their surroundings as the weeks progressed. Finally, the awe walkers experienced increased positive emotions, including more compassion, gratitude and happiness, while feeling less anxious, stressed and depressed.

The experience of awe has been beautifully described by psychologist Dacher Keltner in his recent book *Awe: The Transformative Power of Everyday Wonder*. He explains how experiencing even 5 minutes of awe each day can stimulate curiosity about philosophy, poetry, people, art and life's existential questions. Experiencing awe supports us in building connections with people and the natural world, providing a deeper sense of meaning. Awe is not related to material possessions, technology or status symbols; it exists on a different plane, far away from the everyday world of endless consumerism.

Awe is also felt in moments of collective effervescence – the sense of togetherness experienced at sporting events, celebrations and even funerals. It can be found in the beauty of the built environment, in the cycle of life, in epiphanies and in spiritual experiences. Awe is experienced by witnessing the moral courage, kindness or resilience of others through music, film or art.

When you experience awe, positive neurochemicals like oxytocin and dopamine are released into your system. Oxytocin promotes openness to others and helps you recharge from stress by moving you away from a fight-or-flight state, while dopamine stimulates exploration and wonder. Awe is also associated with lower inflammation, as measured by the biomarker interleukin-6.[2]

Awe is associated with reduced activation of something called the default mode network (or DMN), an area of the brain concerned with self-reflection. This can reduce ruminations associated with depression.[3] As you engage more fully with your surroundings, your mind is not empty or devoid of activity; the prefrontal cortex, the seat of thoughtful analysis in your brain, simply gets a well-deserved 'brain break'. This allows you to move away from the stressed state of busyness and doing towards a state of being.[4]

How do you feel after experiencing a powerful performance in the theatre, viewing a piece of art or spending time in an environment of stunning architecture? Inspired, invigorated, awe-struck even? If so, you are not alone. The brilliant book *Your Brain on Art: How the Arts Transform Us*, written by Susan Magsamen and Ivy Ross, describes how even brief exposure to the broader arts is a health-enhancing experience that can bring transformative wellbeing benefits. Irrespective of your ability level, engaging with any of a wide range of arts activities – whether painting, poetry, performance, creative writing, music or dance – for as little as 45 minutes lowers cortisol.

Research by Daisy Fancourt in University College London has found that people experience significantly higher life satisfaction in terms of mental wellbeing and quality of life when exposed to art-related activities at least once a week, or when attending a cultural event at least once a year. Furthermore, experiencing just one arts activity a month can enhance the quality of your everyday lived experience and enable you to live longer. Exposure to the arts just a couple of times a year can reduce early mortality risk by 14 per cent, whereas more regular exposure can reduce it by 31 per cent. Overall, exposure to the arts may extend your life by up to 10 years.[5]

Awe can be found in the simplest of places. Small micromoments of awe, perhaps just a minute or two each day, enrich your emotional bank account of positivity, enabling more social connection, encouraging kindness and enhancing your wellbeing, lowering inflammation and your stress response while increasing oxytocin.

In terms of mindset, awe can broaden your perspective and worldview as a catalyst that enables you to grow, sometimes in seeking new landscapes but, more importantly, in seeing with new eyes. Awe builds connection to self, to others, to your higher power and to timeless principles of simplicity, universal compassion and radical humility. It is a real win-win-win for you, for others and for the world at large. Can you make some time to experience awe today or this week? It's something your future self will thank you for.

HOW TO INCREASE AWE IN YOUR EVERYDAY LIFE

Being: Be present in the moment to emergent experience. Be more still, more open and curious about the beauty of the world around you.

Seeing: Look upon nature, from vast vistas of mountains or oceans to something minuscule (a variegated leaf or the petal of a flower). View stunning architecture or artwork. Take photographs of what inspires you and review them often. Watch a documentary about the natural world.

Listening: Enjoy birdsong, beautiful music or inspiring words.

Sharing: See a live concert or sporting event with friends, exercise together or share magical moments that create memories.

Witnessing: Witness a child's first steps or a baby's smile, a beautiful sunset, people's extraordinary achievements, kindness or the moral courage of volunteers.

Beat burnout

Do you feel emotionally exhausted and low on energy lately? Do you feel overworked, undervalued and extra cynical? Do you find it hard to switch off? If so, you may be experiencing symptoms of burnout.

Burnout – or occupational burnout, to give it its full name – is now reaching epidemic proportions in the corporate Western world. According to the American Psychology Association's 2023 'Work in America' Survey, 57 per cent of workers said they experienced work-related stress associated with burnout, with negative impacts including emotional exhaustion, irritability and anger.[1]

Of course, burnout exists outside of the modern office or high-stress environments such as busy hospital emergency departments. Consider the person who hasn't had a proper break for years: the mother caring for an ageing parent or a child with disabilities. Caring is wearing, after all. Remember the many people for whom burnout is suffered in silence, taking the form of a gradual disengagement from life itself.

Burnout is now also thought to impact a growing number of carers and caring professionals, including doctors. In the medical and healthcare community, those professionals who are more caring and empathetic are most vulnerable. Documented rates of burnout among health professionals vary but research suggests that it is increasing among doctors since the pandemic.[2]

Of course, the term 'burnout' has been around for quite a while, coined by Herbert Freudenberger in his 1974 book *Burnout: The High Cost of High Achievement*. The medical community was initially reluctant to formally acknowledge the existence of burnout, implying it was, at best, a form of depression in disguise or, at worst, a form of manipulative malingering. However, this is no longer the case, with occupational burnout now officially recognised by the World Health Organisation since 2019.

WHAT EXACTLY IS BURNOUT?

Definition: A syndrome conceptualised as resulting from chronic workplace stress that has not been successfully managed. It is characterised by three dimensions:

1. Feelings of energy depletion or exhaustion
2. Increased mental distance from one's job or feelings of negativity or cynicism related to one's job
3. Reduced professional efficacy.

Burnout refers specifically to phenomena in the occupational context and should not be applied to describe experiences in other areas of life.

While all sources of toxic stress can have a negative impact, burnout is work-related and results from long-standing situational stress that hasn't been managed effectively, either by the individual or by the organisation.

Everyone has challenges in their work and career, and very little is plain sailing. I'm sure you've had times when you have felt overly stressed and underappreciated. Such temporary ups and downs are part and parcel of life itself. However, burnout is different; bad days become the new norm, with prominent feelings of emotional exhaustion and flatness, cynicism and disengagement. As an 'occupational syndrome', burnout has a spectrum of physical, emotional, psychological and relationship symptoms that vary in severity, from mildly disruptive to what I would term a 'full-blown burn', spilling over to impact your relationships, happiness and every aspect of your life.

Physical symptoms can overlap with other symptoms of chronic toxic stress and may include frequent headaches, abdominal cramps or bloating, changes in sleep patterns or eating habits, recurring colds and feeling tired all the time. More long-term adverse physical effects of chronic burnout can increase susceptibility to a range of chronic health conditions, from heart disease and high blood pressure to diabetes and depression.

Emotional symptoms include feeling emotionally 'flat'. An analogy I use is that of a car, with the tyres losing pressure until they are flat. The emotional bank account becomes empty. You may feel you have lost your inner spark of positivity or creative expression. This can lead to emotional exhaustion – feeling dull, listless and wiped out, with simply nothing left to give. As you lose your zest for life, your emotional wellbeing dips.

Mentally, burnout can lead to poor concentration, reduced focus and attention span, and a narrowed sense of perspective. As the amygdala in your brain is on high alert, keeping you in a chronically stressed, fight-or-flight state, you experience diminished productivity and creativity. Your mindset changes, with challenges seeming bleak and insurmountable. You may see tasks you previously found manageable as overwhelming or overly dull, leading to procrastination or simply taking a lot longer to get things done. Negativity about work-related tasks can lead to feelings of cynicism and resentment. Job satisfaction is naturally greatly diminished, with a reduced sense of accomplishment or achievement. This may result in work avoidance or absenteeism.

A lack of confidence, with feelings of self-doubt and difficulty coping, can lead to a sense of failure and futility. You may feel 'trapped', which reduces realistic optimism, or the belief that your situation can change through the power of your own efforts. You become demotivated and less resilient. Overlap with clinical depression may result in symptoms of helplessness, hopelessness and worthlessness, with loss of interest in pleasurable activities. There may even be suicidal thoughts. However, burnout is distinguished from depression (which incorporates negative thoughts, feelings and low mood about all aspects of life, not just work) in that the symptoms of burnout are specifically work-related.

While technology has opened up a whole new world of possibilities in terms of remote working, there is a significant potential downside in that employees can feel that they are literally never away from work. I met a person recently who described how, after a long-distance flight, she opened her iPhone to find that more than 200 emails had landed in her inbox during her 8-hour flight. Little wonder then that she described feelings of 'digital burnout'.

If you are experiencing burnout, you may see a negative impact on your relationships. You may become detached, withdrawn and increasingly isolated as you move back more and more into your own shell, retreating rather than reaching out for support. You may become increasingly irritable and feel resentful towards colleagues and management. Under the dark cloud of burnout, everything looks grim, and it can be hard to have enough energy to care for yourself. Self-care is therefore, more often than not, neglected. An analogy I like to use is that of a wet sponge. With burnout, the sponge is progressively squeezed drier and drier until there is not a drop of effort left to give. Burnout drains the individual of resilience and gradually depletes their reserves in terms of their emotions, mind, body and relationships. To paraphrase Hemingway, burnout happens twice: first, it creeps up gradually, until all of a sudden it hits you instantly.

The bottom line is this – if you are starting to feel emotionally depleted and physically exhausted from your

THINGS YOUR FUTURE SELF WILL THANK YOU FOR

work, becoming detached, disillusioned and cynical, then you may well be on the path to burnout.

Brian was a quiet, somewhat reserved man in his late 30s whom I rarely saw in my medical practice. His last visit had been several years earlier following an ankle injury sustained while jogging on rough terrain. He was married, mortgaged and confidently making his way as a financial analyst in the corporate world.

Then one day I received an urgent call from Brian's father, whom I knew from local sporting circles.

'Can Brian see you today, Mark?' he asked. 'He's in a bad way. We're all very worried about him.'

Two hours later, Brian sat in front of me with a facial expression frozen and devoid of emotion. He was a long way from the jovial young man I remembered. The tears began to flow as he opened up, saying that he couldn't 'take it anymore'. 'It' meant the sleepless nights, chronic stress and constant worrying about work. A year prior, a new senior manager had taken over Brian's team. Their personalities had clashed from the outset and the pressure had become relentless.

'I've always been a hard worker,' Brian told me. 'I used to love my job, but now it's just impossible. No matter how hard I work, it's never enough. I get emails around the clock. Two members of my team left and have not been replaced, so we're under resourced. I also feel I've been unfairly treated by my new manager. Last month she undermined me on a Zoom call in front of the global head of finance and twice she has overlooked me for a promotion. It has made me feel so cynical and disillusioned.'

As I gently probed, Brian shared with me his feelings of emptiness, emotional exhaustion and ennui. 'When I opened the laptop this morning, I felt crushed,' he admitted. 'I just can't do it anymore.'

Brian was hitting the point of full-blown burnout. What started out as a powerful commitment to his career had morphed into a morass of misery. Drop by drop, day by day, his reserves of wellbeing and resilience had been depleted until he had been squeezed dry.

More than anything, Brian felt like a failure, weighed down with guilt and overwhelm. His self-confidence and self-worth had both been slowly eroded. Recent sleepless nights and a mind preoccupied by ruminative negative thoughts had pushed him to the point of exhaustion. My first priority was to remove Brian from his work environment by giving him a medical certificate stating that he was unfit for work. This actually took some considerable persuasion on my part as Brian believed it would ultimately be held against him. Eventually, with the encouragement of his partner, he agreed.

Brian's burnout wasn't fatal or the final straw for his career – far from it. But it was a major wake-up call for him in terms of how he took care of himself, including how he allowed others to treat him. Talk therapy with a trained therapist really helped Brian in this regard, giving him some skills and strategies to see things differently.

As a more active participant in his own wellbeing, he learned the fundamental importance of lifestyle as medicine and taking good care of himself, including being able to switch off and disconnect from work. Brian set some personal self-care goals to help with his burnout recovery; he also found my mindful breathing exercise, PAUSE, very helpful (and see page 195 for a detailed description of it). 'It gave me a very simple way to instantly recharge from stress that only took a minute or two, max. It was a brilliant reminder to actively recharge throughout the day, especially when I didn't feel I needed to.'

Over the course of a few months, Brian became better and stronger and eventually returned to work. He had learned the importance of asking for, and receiving, appropriate resources for projects in the workplace. More importantly, he learned that it wasn't a sign of weakness to ask for help.

Brian's burnout became a breakthrough of sorts for him. He grew enormously as a person in terms of managing his own health and managing himself. He has now become a real leader in his own wellbeing and a powerful advocate for burnout prevention.

As you read this, you may be thinking that Brian's situation doesn't apply to you. However, no matter what field your work is in or what kind of demands it places on you, everyone has a tipping point. This is why I believe it is so important to protect yourself, especially when you believe you don't need to.

Preventing burnout at an organisational level requires that sustainable wellbeing become a key cultural value of the organisation. My advice to employers and managers is to identify those things that matter most to your employees using open forums of communication that safely allow people to be heard. Commit to continually valuing your people by taking small, sustainable steps to make things better. Actions speak louder than words.

My advice for anyone at risk of burnout is simply to become more aware of the potential for it to develop, particularly as it tends to come on gradually and can creep up on you. Awareness precedes change, and paying attention to the early subtle symptoms and signs is so important for your health and wellbeing. If you have some early symptoms of burnout, then a stitch in time may save nine. Invest in self-renewal strategies by taking short breaks during the day, including regular 'circuit breakers' from stress: get out for a short walk in nature, perform a random act of kindness, take a coffee break or have a chat with a friend. Embrace positive lifestyle habits, including regular exercise, restorative sleep and a really nutritious diet. Pay into your emotional bank account by creating a list of the simple things that bring you joy. Perhaps a relaxing bath, a walk in the woods with your best friend or watching a good movie.

Reverse the damage caused by burnout by reaching out to others for support. This includes both support at work and a supportive network outside of work. Disconnect from the overwhelming tsunami of workplace emails during your downtime and instead use that time to recharge and reconnect with others and yourself. Spend quality time with friends and family. Value your human connections and stay connected to causes or community organisations that matter to you. Spending some time alone can also help to bring you more clarity, creativity and confidence.

Finally, reframe your job description. There is always some value to be found in your work. Focus on the aspects you enjoy and you can control. Discover how you can use your strengths at work and how your work can serve and support others. Choosing to change your attitude and mindset about your work can help you regain a sense of purpose in your work life.

Burnout can be prevented and successfully treated. Many of the ideas expressed in this book will support you to do just that. People like Brian are living testament to the capacity to grow stronger from adversity, with a new sense of life purpose and newfound appreciation for well-being. It's never too late to take positive action. If you or someone you know is struggling, remember to reach out for support. You can recover from burnout, restore your equilibrium and rediscover your sparkle.

Avoid 'destination happiness'

Can you take a few minutes to think about the little things that truly make you happy? Many people, when asked what they want from life, will list material successes – a good job, new car, nice house, etc. However, when all the trappings of life are stripped away, more than anything else people tend to seek happiness and fulfilment. Easier said than done, though, given that happiness is a term frequently misunderstood and loaded with misconceptions that, in themselves, can drive so much unhappiness and feelings of inadequacy.

Happiness is often mistaken for a destination – as in, 'I'll be happy when...' When you gain the promotion, recognition, or reward? When you make more money? When you get those new clothes or designer handbag? Or when you're successful – or seen as such by others – having attained whatever it is you believe will make you happy? 'I'll be happy when' is the idea that, right now, in this moment, you are deficient and lacking in some way, which will be made up for by the new possession or achievement. Given there is always something else to attain, working towards 'destination happiness' means always being somewhat dissatisfied with the here and now. This leading to discontentment, negative comparison, and a sense of scarcity – 'chronic not-enoughness.' This mindset can trigger feelings of anxiety and toxic stress, while taking away from your ability to be present and simply enjoy the moment.

Societal pressure, particularly from social media, can be a major cause of this, creating a fear of missing out or 'FOMO', and fostering feelings of inadequacy, envy or jealousy. It can also set an unrealistic bar for achievement, resulting in blame and self-recrimination when you inevitably fall short of reaching the stars.

Now don't get me wrong, achievement and success can be a tremendous source of fulfilment. There's nothing wrong with setting and working toward great goals or with having nice things. Just don't expect them to bring you lasting happiness on their own.

There's an old Eastern fable about the Buddha and one of his students.

'More than anything, I want happiness,' the student proclaims to his master. 'But how can I find it?'

'It's easy and difficult at the same time, requiring only two tasks from you,' replied the wise teacher. 'Firstly, remove "I", which represents your untamed ego of entitlement and expectation. Secondly, let go of "want", the root of desire which fuels so much unhappiness. Now, my friend, having let go of "I" and "want", you are left with "happiness"!'

Of course, I'm not suggesting it's possible to be happy all the time, as real life provides plenty of setbacks and speed bumps. In Buddhist philosophy, there can be no real happiness without, at some point, experiencing its opposite – suffering. Suffering and happiness are seen as two sides of the same coin. The bittersweet paradox of joy means that, without the pain of separation, it is impossible to fully experience the joy of reunion; without the pain of effort, it is impossible to fully experience the joy of reward; without the pain of rejection, it is impossible to fully experience the joy of acceptance.

Destination happiness is the false narrative that a happy life equates to a flawless flow of positive emotions and successes while never experiencing negative emotions. Negative emotions such as fear, anger, anxiety and guilt are a very real part of being human and are not meant to be denied, suppressed or repressed. Give yourself permission to be more human by making the best of good times, with the resilience to embrace defeat, disappointments and tough times. This is the very essence of emotional agility – becoming more curious about the source of negative emotions rather than trying to suppress them by sweeping them under the carpet.

Flourishing in life is about creating a ratio of positive to negative emotions of at least three to one. Many people experience a ratio of perhaps two or two-and-a-half to one; good things going on, but with a downward drag of negative emotion as well. Getting this 'positivity ratio' above three to one can create a tipping point for wellbeing, which broadens and builds your capacity to flourish both in your personal and professional life.

There is clearly a difference between your moment-to-moment experience of happiness right now as you read this and your sense of reflected happiness when you look back at how happy and satisfied you are with your life overall. In general sustainable happiness is made up of some key 'ingredients': pleasure and positive emotions, engagement, relationships, meaning and accomplishments. This model of wellbeing, known as PERMA, was devised by American psychologist Martin Seligman to describe the various elements that individually and in combination support an emotionally flourishing life.

Pleasure and positive emotions

The subjective experience of positive emotion includes feelings of love, optimism, excitement, enthusiasm, joy or gratitude. While fleeting in nature, positive emotions provide temporary sparks of happiness. Experiencing pleasure is a profound psychological need. This makes sense as we are all pleasure (not pain!) seekers. Compared to the long-lasting effects that negative emotion has, positive emotion is generally temporary and transient – otherwise, your brain would adapt and turn pleasure into routine. However, it can still be powerful when it comes to enhancing your wellbeing.

Positive emotion about the present moment can be enhanced by greater awareness of the now and by savouring physical pleasures; positive emotion about the future can be enhanced by cultivating hope and optimism; and positive emotion about past events can be increased through building the habits of gratitude and forgiveness.

Engagement

Having a strong sense of engagement is essentially experiencing a feeling of flow. Flow is a universal psychological experience characterised by being engaged and energised, with a deep feeling of enjoyment. It is experienced when you apply your skills to a challenging activity in pursuit of a clear goal. Self-awareness disappears as concentration is fully absorbed in the present moment, detached from the stresses of the past or future. With immediate feedback on progress, feelings of flow can be immensely gratifying, with the activity itself being its own reward. Many people experience flow in seemingly simple life situations such as driving the car, cooking, studying, gardening, engaging in creative pursuits or even carrying out a satisfying work task. Perhaps you even feel it when you are engaged in a conversation with friends. Creating flow experiences in your life can be a gateway to real inner happiness; a valuable tool in the creation of a more productive and rewarding life.

Relationships

Sustainable happiness doesn't occur in a vacuum – it requires human connection. Strong, supportive inter-personal relationships are the leading indicator of your wellbeing and enable you to experience more happiness as a byproduct of being listened to, valued, supported and understood. Feelings of togetherness, connection and community enhance your happiness and wellbeing. By contrast, loneliness and isolation can lead to so much unhappiness, with a detrimental impact on your wellbeing.

Meaning

Sustainable happiness also requires a sense of meaning, enabling you to transcend setbacks and life challenges to connect with a bigger why.

One of the keys to a life of fulfilment and meaning is to have a strong sense of purpose. This includes both inner purpose (or a sense of being – the feeling that life is worth living) and outer purpose (or a sense of doing – the source of value in your life that is worth living for). In other words, purpose for you while also providing benefit for others. Purpose can act as a catalyst for enhanced wellbeing, generating feelings of happiness and fulfilment while creating a ripple effect of contagious positivity throughout your life.

Accomplishments

Bettering yourself, succeeding, setting and working towards goals consistent with your values can help to foster a sense of accomplishment essential to happiness. William Butler Yeats, one of the world's greatest poets, once wrote that happiness is neither pleasure nor virtue nor this nor that, but simply growth. We are happiest when we are growing, climbing a mountain of value to us, neither necessarily reaching the summit nor wandering aimlessly at the foothills. In other words, connecting to a cause bigger than yourself.

Many people pursue a sense of mastery and achievement, whether in terms of academics, career, sport or
hobbies. This 'accomplishing life' can provide a tremendous amount of life satisfaction, often when achieved
simply for its own sake independent of any external reward.

To the five areas of PERMA I would add health in a
holistic sense and really valuing your own self-care needs
in terms of mind, body, emotion and spirit. As a medical
doctor, my interest in the science of more sustainable
happiness and wellbeing boils down to this key essential
fact: being happier and more fulfilled can improve your
health in so many ways.

Firstly, feeling happy releases a number of positivity
neurochemicals that not only boost feelings of wellbeing
but diminish stress hormones and support neuroplasticity.
You boost your own emotional bank account so that you
have a reservoir of positivity to draw upon when you need
it. Being happier also helps to increase vagal tone, which
improves the functionality of the vagus nerves. The vagus
nerves are the longest nerves in the body, winding their way
from the brain stem all the way to the gut. They provide
constant connection and communication between the
heart, brain and gut, forming what is known as the parasympathetic nervous system. This is the opposite of the
fight-or-flight stress response that occurs with activation

of the sympathetic nervous system and is important for stress recharge. The vagus nerves are involved with regulation of blood pressure, heart rate, speech, taste, mucus production in lungs, digestion, mood, frequency of urination, breathing rate, immune response, skin and muscle sensations amongst others. Its functions are more easily remembered though the terms 'pause and plan', 'feed and breed' or 'rest and digest'.

Feeling happier opens your mind to seeing the world through the lens of more abundance and appreciation, supporting resilience and a sense of realistic optimism. This more open mindset boosts your imagination and strengthens innovation as you see things more creatively and expansively. As all learning has an emotional base, when you feel happier you learn more effectively and boost your memory. You become better able to embrace positive change in your life, boosting willpower and supporting healthier habits.

What's more, feeling happier has been found to be contagious. Research by Nicholas Christakis in Yale University has highlighted how happiness can spread outwards to three degrees of separation. In fact, each happy friend you have can increase your happiness by 9 per cent while each unhappy friend can reduce your happiness by 7 per cent.[1]

The prevailing mindset nowadays is that life success leads to happiness. While there is no doubt that achievements and accomplishments can provide feelings of immense satisfaction, embracing happiness in the moment – no matter where we are at with our personal goals – can lead to even greater accomplishments and more sustainable success in the future. This new paradigm is the polar opposite of destination happiness and holds true whether you define sustainable success by your relationships, achievements, performance, creativity, energy or your health.

The bluebird represents hope, springtime renewal and happiness in many cultures. An early-20th-century Belgian play called *The Blue Bird* epitomises for me the essence of what it means to pursue happiness as an elusive destination. It describes the adventures of two young children, Mytyl and her brother Tyltyl, who leave their home in the woods to find the bluebird of happiness. They travel the world in vain searching for the bluebird, eventually arriving back home to discover that the blue bird had been right there all along.

Many of us can fall victim to the destination happiness mindset, and as a result, end up looking for happiness in all the wrong places. Get off the treadmill to 'destination happiness' by letting go of the need to be perfect – life is never perfect for anyone so don't expect perfection from yourself. Learn to embrace your flaws, make peace with the past, live more in the present moment, accept what you can't change and find the courage to change what you can. Let go of negative comparison, the thief of joy. Work on accepting yourself for who you are and treating yourself with self-compassion.

One of my favourite interviews I have done for my podcast to date has been with Zara King, a journalist and well-known Irish media personality. She gives off an air of infectious optimism and positivity, borne out by her evident bubbly personality. When asked about the meaning of life, she answered, 'To love and be loved as a fair, kind and decent human being.'

What struck me most, though, were her wise words about the negative impact society's attitude to happiness is having on so many people, particularly younger people. Her advice was to 'reframe your happiness to the here and now. Set goals, certainly, but don't bank your happiness on simply achieving them as that can weigh you down. As an eternal optimist I'm a great believer that what you put out in the world comes back, so when you put positivity in your life it comes back to you. Appreciate you can make happiness an everyday choice; focus on what you have, the little things.' I couldn't agree more!

Everyone has their own journey in life and there is no one-size-fits-all approach to health or happiness. As a concept, happiness is not something you can pursue; rather, it is the byproduct of doing something that connects you with others or helps someone else, provides pleasure or purposeful engagement or feelings of flow, connection or fulfilment. That's why my favourite definition of happiness is having someone to love and care for, something to be grateful for, something useful to do and something to look forward to.

Appreciate the many different ways that you can enhance your inner feelings of happiness and contentment, from gratitude and giving to presence and purpose. Just as Mytyl and Tyltyl learned, the bluebird of happiness might be right under your nose if you choose to see him more clearly. Rather than a destination, happiness can be a choice that you make every day. You can choose presence, peace and contentment, to value the ordinary and everyday, the very gift that is life itself.

Learn to PAUSE

The ever-accelerating pace of modern life and the real pressures that come with it mean that mindfulness has never been more necessary. Even without distress or immediate distractions, it's amazing how easy it can be to miss what's right in front of you. With so much distracted doing, finding even a few moments to rest in being can be a real challenge.

This tendency to avoid the full experience of 'the now' is unfortunate because, whether it's a busy weekday or a relaxing weekend, and whether you feel calm or anxious, tired or energised, serene or stressed, the now is all you have. The present moment is all any of us have. Life unfolds for each of us, one breath, one moment, and one day at a time. It's easy to become weighed down by heaviness, toxic stress and needless negativity, which can pull you away from your true self. This was my own experience many years ago, when a 'perfect storm' of life events, including bereavements and business pressures, made me realise that I needed a pathway to sustainable presence and peaceful equanimity. As a result, I found mindfulness – or rather, mindfulness found me.

Mindfulness is the practice of paying attention, on purpose, in the present moment. It includes the principles of patience, awareness, acceptance, letting go, not judging, not striving, trust and seeing things as if for the first time.

Dr Herbert Benson was a pioneering leader in the emerging field of mind-body medicine. His ideas about the link between stress and ill health were so revolutionary in the 1950s that he allegedly had to conduct his experiments at night to avoid attention and potential backlash from more conservative medical colleagues. He suggested that most healthcare visits were related to stress-induced conditions.

As a heart specialist, he observed two key things: first, that stress-related behaviours negatively impacted risk factors for heart disease; and second, that activating what he called the 'relaxation response' by stimulating the parasympathetic nervous system could reduce this risk. He went on to found and direct the Benson-Henry Institute for Mind-Body Medicine at Harvard-affiliated Massachusetts General Hospital. Meeting and hearing him speak in Boston a few years before he passed away was a career highlight for me. His authentic nature, calm demeanour and ability to communicate complex ideas with simplicity left a lasting impression.

Herbert Benson's work focused on eliciting the relaxation response through two simple steps. Firstly, by repeating a word, phrase or sound – for example, gently saying the word 'peace' with each exhale. Alternatively, one could repeat a phrase like 'I am peace', saying 'I am' while inhaling and 'peace' while exhaling. Secondly, and most importantly, gently and intentionally returning to this word or phrase whenever your mind becomes distracted by other thoughts.

The essence of the relaxation response is that it acts as a circuit breaker for the constant stream of everyday thoughts. It becomes an antidote to feelings of toxic stress, overwhelm or the anxious ruminations of your merry-go-mind – that endless carousel of negative thoughts that can take over your brain. It can be a powerful tool when you feel disconnected from your true self.

The relaxation response not only feels good, but it also offers significant health benefits. Although these

ideas originated thousands of years ago in Eastern tradi-
tions, they were initially dismissed in the West as 'voodoo
medicine' and not seen as real science. Thanks in large
part to pioneering research by people like Herbert Benson
and Jon Kabat-Zinn, recent years have seen a surge of
research highlighting the health benefits of mindfulness
in managing conditions ranging from high blood pressure to irritable bowel syndrome.[1] Research conducted at
Harvard University and Massachusetts General Hospital
used fMRI scans to examine the brains of participants in
mind-body medicine programmes. They found that eight
weeks of mindfulness-based stress reduction (MBSR)
led to changes in the brain, strengthening areas associated with the sense of self, perspective, learning, memory
and emotional regulation.[2] Meanwhile, the amygdala, the
brain's emotional alarm centre, became less prominent – a
change correlated with reduced perceived stress. MBSR
programmes can enhance present-moment experience
while reducing the influence of the 'narrative network',
the story of who you believe you are.[3]

Breathing is key to the relaxation response. Unlike
mouth breathing, research has shown that breathing
through your nose helps synchronise activity in brain areas
like the olfactory cortex, amygdala, and hippocampus.
This supports recovery from stress and helps manage
anxiety.[4] To quote the poet Rumi, 'There is one way of

breathing that is constricted and shameful. Then, there's another way: a breath of love that takes you all the way to infinity.'

Everyone has the ability to tap into the relaxation response. If you practise yoga, you may have already done this through practices like yoga nidra, often done at the end of a class. If not, here is a simple guide on how to elicit the relaxation response yourself at home. It only requires a few minutes of your time – ideally about ten.

Begin by finding a comfortable position, either sitting or lying down, in a quiet place free from interruptions. It's best not to set an alarm, as you might spend the time anticipating when it will go off. Relax your body, close your eyes and focus on your breath. Inhale slowly and steadily through your nose, paying attention to how the air moves through your nostrils and expands your lungs. As you exhale, silently say a word or phrase that feels natural to you. This could be a general word like 'peace' or 'love', or a phrase that comes naturally to you. If you practise a particular religion, you might find a line or phrase that resonates with your beliefs. For example, a Buddhist might say 'Om', while a Catholic might repeat 'Hail Mary, full of grace'. Continue to gently repeat your chosen word or phrase for about ten minutes, and then allow your thoughts to return naturally. Open your eyes and rest in presence in a seated position for a moment or two.

Understanding the many benefits of mindful breathing and inspired by the work of Herbert Benson, I decided to simplify this practice for use in my everyday medical practice with patients. This led me to develop the 1-minute PAUSE technique, offering a quick entry point into mindfulness and mind-body medicine.

THE PAUSE TECHNIQUE

P: Pause

Take a break from whatever you're doing, just for a moment.

A: Awareness and Attention

Notice how you're feeling physically and mentally. You might feel stressed or anxious, or perhaps you notice tension in your shoulders. Simply observe and feel these sensations in your body and mind, not just intellectually but also emotionally and physically. Don't try to explain or rationalise your feelings; just witness and give them attention.

U: Understanding

Understand and appreciate that you are separate from your feelings. Like observing a flowing river, you are merely observing your feelings of stress or anxiety. They are not who you are.

S: Simply Breathe

Take a slow, deep breath in, from the top of your nose to the bottom of your lungs, and hold it briefly.

E: Exhale

Exhale fully and steadily through your nostrils, emptying your lungs. As you exhale, release all your tension, toxic stress and anxiety. Let it go, then pause briefly before repeating the exercise.

By practising four or five deep breaths like this over the course of a minute, you create a quick and sustainable self-care strategy that can immediately disrupt stress. Many people find that reclaiming their attention through their breath calms stress and anxiety while fostering a peaceful presence.

As you slow your breathing and your heart rate decreases, you stimulate your parasympathetic nervous system, which governs relaxation and is controlled by the vagus nerve. The vagus nerve acts like an information superhighway, sending neurochemical signals between the brain and body, enabling recovery from stress. Mindful breathing has been shown to reduce cellular inflammation, with positive effects on both telomeres and biological ageing.

Slow, deep breaths can also increase heart rate variability (HRV). This is the gap between your heart rate when you inhale (which is slightly higher) and when you exhale (which is slightly lower). Higher HRV is associated with a more finely tuned vagal response, helping you recharge from stress.

Teaching mindful breathing required me to first become comfortable and confident with the practice myself, moving beyond merely knowing the theory and benefits. I began embodying the practice through daily action. I placed Post-it notes with the word PAUSE all around me – on the bathroom mirror, at my computer, in the car. These reminders helped me to internalise the practice. PAUSE shifted from being an interesting health tool to becoming part of my heart and mind.

While you can simply focus on breathing during PAUSE, I, like Herbert Benson, prefer to focus on words. Here's an example of using a positive word on the inhale and a negative word on the exhale, helping restore emotional balance:

> *As I breathe in courage, I breathe out fear.*
> *As I breathe in calm, I breathe out anxiety.*
> *As I breathe in peace, I breathe out anger.*
> *As I breathe in self-care, I breathe out self-neglect.*
> *As I breathe in serenity, I breathe out stress.*

I soon began teaching PAUSE to patients, starting with those dealing with toxic stress or overwhelm, and eventually offering it as a general self-care strategy for enhanced wellbeing.

The beauty of PAUSE lies in its simplicity. Sixty seconds for self-care is such a small commitment, making it immediately achievable. From this starting point, you can extend the practice as long as you'd like. In my wellness workshops, the extended version lasts nearly 10 minutes.

PAUSE offers a path of progressive self-awareness, allowing you to step out of mindlessness and into mindful presence. It helps realign and balance your inner and outer worlds with peace, gentleness and harmony. By consciously redirecting your attention to your breath, you shift from the constant busyness of doing to the simplicity of being, making room for the present moment.

PAUSE creates space for stillness, simplicity and serenity. It invites self-care and self-compassion, fostering a state of calm, presence and hope. Through the relaxation response you reconnect with your true self, experiencing more inner peace, contentment and a deeper sense of who you are. This opens the door to life's inherent richness, allowing you to live more fully, moment by moment, with presence.

Unplug with forest therapy

Have you spent any time in nature recently? With more people than ever living in urban environments, it has never been easier to feel separated from nature and the natural world. Despite this unfortunate reality, our natural state is to be deeply connected with nature. Scientific research highlights that spending 2 hours per week in nature will lower stress and enhance your health and overall well-being.[1] Forest therapy is an opportunity to rediscover nature and, in doing so, rediscover and reconnect with yourself.

As a long-time advocate of the many health-enhancing benefits of spending time in nature, a question I'm often asked is how to 'do' forest therapy. It's a great question.

Forest therapy, as a multisensory immersion in the natural world, has less to do with doing and is more about being – being fully and mindfully present during an immersive experience with nature. No more, no less. Mindful presence means exactly that – consciously choosing to be present where you are when you're there, fully and completely.

Forest therapy is about fostering a deeper connection with the natural world by disconnecting from the busyness and distractions of everyday life and reconnecting with the essence of who you are. In essence, it is the practice of immersing yourself in nature using all five senses. This enables you to connect with the natural world in a more immersive way and to enjoy its therapeutic benefits. To be completely clear, forest therapy is not intended to replace professional medical advice, treatment or counselling for those who are unwell. It works best as part of a holistic approach to self-care to recharge from stress, re-energise, and enhance your wellbeing.

As a therapeutic tool, forest therapy – also known as forest bathing – started in Japan in 1982 with research on Japanese businessmen. The group studied were prone to overwork, with all of the associated toxic stress and negative health consequences. In fact, there is even a term for death by overwork in Japan – *karoshi*. The research found that time spent in nature could significantly lower levels of the stress hormone cortisol and reduce blood pressure while increasing vigour and vitality. The health-enhancing benefits of time spent in nature deservedly attracted serious attention. Eventually, it led to the adoption of the term 'forest bathing' or *shinrin-yoku*, from the Japanese words 'shinrin' meaning forest and 'yoku' meaning bath.

By 'bathing' in the essence of the forest and engaging with the natural rhythm of nature, you allow yourself to relax and recharge from stress in a way that supports harmony and healing.

What's really interesting is that only a very small percentage (perhaps as little as 5 per cent) of your brain's activity is at the level of conscious perception, with the rest below this level of conscious awareness. Just as only a small percentage of an iceberg is visible, with the vast majority hidden underwater, similarly, you may be consciously unaware of up to 95 per cent of your brain's cognitive inputs. This is why it can be so easy to underestimate the substantial benefits of time spent in health-enhancing environments such as nature.

Let's explore how some aspects of a forest therapy experience can boost your health, wellbeing and vitality.

Spending time in nature increases your degree of emotional positivity, boosting subjective wellbeing and happiness. You may feel more enthusiastic and hopeful, with a boost in mood as you may enter a flow state. Time in nature lowers levels of stress hormones, such as cortisol.

It reduces sympathetic nervous system activity, aka the stressed state, while boosting parasympathetic nervous system activity, which supports recovery from stress. It can increase heart rate variability, a measure of the degree of balance in your nervous system.

Spending time in nature regularly can reduce the risk of many chronic health conditions. It can lower blood pressure and heart rate and improve cardiac health. Time spent regularly in nature can increase your pain threshold, improve biological functions and boost energy, feelings of vigour and vitality.[2] Time in nature also enhances empathy, feelings of compassion and altruism. It strengthens your sense of connection to the natural world, while fostering feelings of awe and transcendence. *Yugen* is a Japanese term that translates as 'mysterious profundity', an intuitive feeling of how nature can encapsulate you in a transcendent way, not easily expressed in words. It is a sort of imaginative sixth sense that enables time in nature to inspire new ideas, boost creativity and shift perspectives.

Being immersed in the wonderful environment of nature supports more mindful presence, which increases attention span, focus and short-term memory. It quietens the merry-go-mind of anxious negative thoughts, reducing feelings of irritability and toxic stress. It can alleviate anxiety and decrease depressive feelings. You become more other-centred: nicer to and more considerate of others. You also develop a stronger sense of self, in terms of self-awareness and self-compassion.

So, here's my guide on how to 'be' with nature through forest therapy, one mindful step at a time.

Step 1: Begin

The beginning of a forest therapy experience is like accepting an invitation – nature's invitation to engage. It's an opportunity to gravitate from the busyness of life to the lightness of the natural world, opening your senses to engage with nature, one breath, one moment and one mindful step at a time.

Clearly, it is not possible to disconnect from the stresses and strains of everyday life if your mobile phone is buzzing in your back pocket. If practical, leave it at home, turn it off or, at the very least, place it on 'silent mode' for the duration of your forest therapy time.

As an idea, you could park any pressing problems or concerns by writing them down in a notebook or journal before you start out. If there is some issue you want to solve, you might set a simple intention as you begin your forest therapy experience in nature. Through conscious immersion in nature, your subconscious mind will continue to work creatively. Perhaps later in the day you will feel inspired and gain fresh insights.

Step 2: Reconnect

Reconnect with the richness of the natural world as you slow down and allow yourself to be still. Immerse yourself in the experience of nature by focusing on your breath and ignoring the noise of your inner thoughts. Ask yourself, what do you see? What do you sense? What do you smell? How do you feel right now? Listen in all directions and focus on what you hear: the wind rustling gently through the trees; birdsong in the distance; the silence beyond that.

For me, a short mindful breathing exercise (see my PAUSE exercise on page 195) is a terrific way to ground myself in awareness and tune in to the present moment. Deep breathing in nature brings fresh oxygen to your cells and can expose you to phytoncides, natural plant substances that can lower inflammation, boost immunity and support wellbeing.

Step 3: Observe

Become the observer of all your experiences through the lens of your senses. Simply notice what you notice, over and over again. Give your analytical mind a break as you tune into your feelings.

Ask yourself how you feel when you:

- hear birdsong or the gentle breeze rustling through the trees?
- see the beautiful fractal patterns of the leaves and trees?
- experience the warm sun at your back?
- feel the breeze against your face?
- sense the crisp crunching of leaves underfoot?
- smell the lush fragrance of the forest?
- taste the fresh forest air?

Become one with nature using your five senses of sound, sight, smell, touch and taste. Walk slowly to keep your senses attuned to your environment. How does your body feel as it moves? If you like, sit down for a while as you simply soak up the sounds, sensations and scenery around you.

Step 4: Listen

Notice the soundscapes of nature and what – or who – made them.

For me, experiencing the sounds of birdsong is one of the highlights of spending time in nature. I find it incredibly peaceful, transporting me to a different realm of relaxation. Maybe it does the same for you too. But birdsong doesn't just instil a feeling of serene pleasure – it has also been scientifically demonstrated to have objective wellbeing benefits. Research highlights how exposure to birdsong can reduce anxiety and irrational thoughts, leading to significant mental health and wellbeing benefits not just for those suffering from depression or anxiety but for healthy individuals too.[3]

Birdsong relaxes the body while boosting brain function. It can support alertness and attention span, cognitive focus and concentration, while also reducing feelings of fatigue.[4] Research has also found that hearing birdsong for as little as 7 minutes can enhance feelings of wellbeing.[5]

Nobody is sure exactly why birdsong can boost wellbeing. Perhaps it is due to birdsong's deep sensory connection with nature or perhaps hearing it triggers a reminder of the positive experiences we have in that environment. Perhaps it's the direct lowering of stress hormone levels such as cortisol, given that from an evolutionary viewpoint, the presence of birdsong may indicate a safer, less threatening environment. Perhaps the sound of birdsong supports 'soft fascination' – a form of attentive awareness which recharges you from feelings of psychological stress and attentional fatigue. This is one of the key benefits of time spent in the natural world, a 'brain break' as it were, restoring attention and allowing you to more fully rest in 'being'.

Recently a study on the effect of birdsong was carried out with almost 1,300 participants. A smartphone app called 'Urban Mind' was used to gather information about their wellbeing and environments three times a day. The research found a significant positive association between mental wellbeing and hearing or seeing birds, even after controlling for other variables such as occupation, education status or factors that can enhance wellbeing (such as time near water or greenery). A lasting benefit from birdsong on mental wellbeing was also demonstrated, meaning that the subjective benefits lasted well beyond the time of exposure to the birdsong itself.

One of birdsong's benefits is its stochastic nature. In other words, it is composed of lots of random sounds with no particular pattern or repetitive rhythm to focus on.

Nature's alarm clock, the dawn chorus, signals the start of a new day while simultaneously stimulating a sense of arousal. At a deeper level, birdsong resonates with feelings of safety and security, with its absence or cessation a sign of potential danger or threat. While one swallow never made a summer, the soundscapes of birdsong do seem to boost your subjective health and mental wellbeing.

Of course, there are many other soundscapes of nature: the wind rustling through the leaves of the trees, the scuffling sound of twigs crunching underfoot. And then there is the particular kind of silence found in nature. *Teanga na Locha* is a beautiful old Irish description of the sound of silence near a lake. It's the silence between notes that creates music and the silence between words that creates language. Similarly, experiencing relative silence in nature, punctuated by a solitary birdsong perhaps, can greatly add to the auditory experience.

Step 5: Look

To paraphrase Marcel Proust, you don't need to seek new landscapes but instead to see with new eyes. With 'new eyes' of presence and openness, what do you now notice? What are your eyes drawn to? What do you see? Are there different shades of green visible, or vistas of speckled sunlight through the leaves?

Observe the intricately designed fractal patterns of nature. Notice the patterns in the flower petals or veins in a leaf.

Can you see how the same view is constantly changing, dependent on the amount of natural light, time of day or season? Can you experience a deepening sense of awe and appreciation of the natural world as you become more attuned to the unfolding fractal patterns that surround you? Can you choose to view everything around you through different eyes, experiencing the bigger picture? Seeing the interconnection of all things opens the doorway to greater knowing and understanding. How does this make you feel?

Step 6: Smell

What do you smell? The soil, plant aromas, phytoncides, the fresh oxygen-rich clean air? 'Petrichor' is the name for that rich, earthy scent that comes when dry ground has been soaked by recent rain. Similarly, freshly cut grass releases several chemicals that stimulate the hippocampus (memory centre) and amygdala, and work to reduce feelings of stress by lowering cortisol levels.

Your nose contains hundreds of scent receptors which can detect about one trillion separate smells. These are stimulated by tiny molecules in your environment that enter your nose and interact with the olfactory epithelium. The olfactory epithelium consists of two patches, each measuring about 5cm^2, located in the roof of the nasal cavities. From here they connect with nerve cells that relay to the olfactory cortex, located in the temporal lobe of the brain. This is a brain area involved in memory and emotion, which is why smells can be so evocative in terms of triggering emotional and physical responses.

Step 7: Touch

What can you touch? How does it feel? Your fingers, hands, toes and feet are very sensitive to minute cues that elicit physiological and emotional responses that can register in the brain within 50 milliseconds.

Put your hands on a tree trunk and feel its rugged presence. Hug it if you wish. As you touch the tree, appreciate that you are part of a bigger whole, part of the bigger mystery of universal consciousness. Pick up some leaves or small stones. If appropriate, remove your socks and shoes to ground down into the earth beneath you. Imagine roots spreading downward from your feet into the ground, plugging you into relaxation and recharging you from stress.

Many people describe subjective wellbeing benefits from this practice of grounding – direct contact with the surface of the Earth with your bare feet or hands. This is thought to enable free electrons from the Earth's surface to spread over and into the body, where they can have antioxidant effects that support immune health, lower cellular inflammation and enhance wellbeing.[6]

Step 8: Taste

What can you taste? This is a sense often forgotten while in nature. Bringing along some fresh berries to eat can provide a wonderful immersive experience. Alternatively, just opening your mouth and sticking your tongue out to taste the forest air (or rain) can deepen your connection with nature.

Step 9: Reflect

Before you leave the space, reflect on all you have noticed. Perhaps you might like to write a few lines in a journal describing your experience with forest therapy. How do you feel now from an emotional viewpoint, compared to beforehand? Mentally more relaxed? Physically more revitalised? How can this experience inform your life going forward?

Several years ago, I had the opportunity to visit the magnificent Muir Woods. Just outside San Francisco, Muir Woods has some of the oldest and biggest Dawn Redwood trees in the world. It's a terrific spot for forest therapy. John Muir, who was one of the great 19th-century pioneering advocates for planting woods and trees, once wrote that 'in every walk with nature, one receives far more than he seeks'.

In that sense, I believe it is important to end with a simple gratitude practice. Giving thanks for participating as the 'noticer' helps to further consolidate the forest bathing experience and deepen your relationship with nature, making you more aware of your senses and how they support your wellbeing, and of how the sights, smells, soundscapes, sensations and tastes of nature have impacted your lived experience today.

Perhaps you are grateful for your mind that allows you to reflect, observe and better understand yourself and others. Grateful for your heart that provides so much empathy and compassion. Grateful for your physical body that enables you to be in the world.

As you breathe, appreciate the fresh oxygen-rich air that is filling your lungs.

End your forest therapy experience grounded in awareness and attuned to the present moment. With your eyes open or closed, breathe slowly and steadily as you inhale the richness of the natural world.

Forest therapy plugs you into the bounty and beauty of nature, recharging from stress, bringing you feelings of serenity and peaceful equanimity. It's a terrific reminder of the security and sheer magnificence that nature provides. Imagine a bridge between you and a future, more vitalised version of yourself. Forest therapy can become that bridge, taking you home not just to nature but to *your* true nature. It's a gateway from distracted doing to being more present in the natural world; a roadway to recharge from stress and revitalise your wellbeing; a pathway to plug you into a bigger connection with the universe. A journey to inner peace.

Your Personal Fulfilment

Lifelong learning provides a stepping stone to a brighter and more meaningful future

Make every day a learning day

When was the last time you learned something new or did something for the first time?

Whenever I consider the benefits of lifelong learning, Bill comes to mind. Bill had spent most of his life working as a cabbie in London until retirement took him home to Ireland at the age of 70.

Bill seemed to have an insatiable thirst for learning, always reading a book whenever I met him at the medical practice. During the Covid lockdowns, he had taken Spanish language lessons online. More recently, he was listening to and learning from a podcast about Irish history.

One day I asked Bill if he'd always had such a great love of learning. He told me that while he hadn't exactly been the top of his class in school, he'd always enjoyed learning about history and geography.

'The toughest test I ever took was the Knowledge,' Bill told me. 'I studied almost every day for three and a half years before I passed the test and got my green badge. For some friends of mine, it took even longer. It was well worth it though. I made a good living from it, but it also gave me a great sense of achievement.'

Curious to learn more, I asked Bill to explain what the world-renowned 'Knowledge test', also known as the Knowledge of London, had involved. To become a licensed taxi driver in London, one must have a thorough knowledge of its geography within a 6-mile radius of Charing Cross. Over 25,000 streets and thousands of place names, land-marks and significant buildings along London's intricate road network must be memorised for taxi drivers to be able to get from point A to point B in the shortest possible time (without Google Maps!). Memorising these 320 distinct routes takes considerable time and effort; mastering the Knowledge typically takes students three to four years. I thought it sounded not unlike medical school with its inti-mate knowledge of human anatomy.

What's really fascinating about the Knowledge test is the impact this acquired knowledge can have on your brain, specifically on the part of the brain dealing with memory, which is known as the hippocampus. Neuroscientists at University College London carried out fMRI scans on the brains of London cab drivers and found that they had larger hippocampi than non-taxi drivers.[1] However, this didn't necessarily prove any association, as it was possible that people with larger hippocampi had simply chosen to become taxi drivers rather than the work itself influencing brain changes. So to investigate further, they scanned the brains of trainee taxi drivers before, during and after their training, subsequently comparing their brain scans with their success in the Knowledge test.

Their findings were incredible. While there was no difference in hippocampus size before the training began, those who successfully completed the Knowledge test were found to have larger hippocampi, highlighting that learning can change the structure of your brain through a process known as neuroplasticity. If ever there was a case for learning, this must surely be it – a bigger brain with better memory that can support you in being more successful and perhaps protect you from age-related memory loss.

But you don't need to become a London taxi driver to experience the brain-boosting benefits of learning. It's all about starting, and the best place to start is in your own mind by adopting a growth mindset approach to learning and to life.

The terms 'fixed mindset' and 'growth mindset' were introduced by American psychologist Carol Dweck and represent the inner beliefs that people have about their potential ability.

The fixed mindset believes that your talent and ability are set in stone and essentially unchangeable through effort or practice. It becomes an all-or-nothing world view which sees failure as a zero-sum game – in other words, you either have it or you don't! Ironically, the fixed mindset may disregard effort too on the grounds that if you were really that good, you wouldn't need to practise. Furthermore, experiencing success with a fixed mindset can lead to impostor syndrome, triggering feelings of inadequacy and insecurity.

On the other hand, a growth mindset sees talent as a starting point, valuing effort and potential improvement. It understands that skills can be developed and improved over time. Rather than obstacles, challenges become opportunities to learn and grow, through a journey of improvement and discovery. Research has shown that teaching about the brain's capacity to change through neuroplasticity can support the growth mindset and act as a catalyst for personal growth. Reframing your world-view through more of a growth mindset can boost grit and resilience, leading to enhanced emotional wellbeing, greater life satisfaction and a path of self-development.[2]

Einstein once famously said that he had no special talent except to be passionately curious. Genuine curiosity is a hallmark of lifelong learners, as it encourages you to keep asking better and more interesting questions. It fosters humility through an appreciation that there is so much to learn and that you don't have all the answers. Curiosity broadens your mindset, enabling you to take different perspectives on board. As such, you deepen awareness, build empathy and strengthen relationships. Curiosity can become a catalyst for personal growth and enhanced wellbeing by creating the conditions for a more interesting and fulfilling life.

Have you ever considered learning a new language? Irrespective of whether this happens when you are aged 17 or 77, research from the University of Edinburgh, published in the *Annals of Neurology*, has found a positive impact on brain ability, especially in terms of reading and general intelligence.

Learning a new language can build new brain capacity in both the cerebral cortex and hippocampus. The cerebral cortex is the master organiser of your brain, involved in perception, attention, awareness and action. Enhancing this can improve focus and attention span, making it easier to avoid distractions while improving the capacity to switch tasks.

The hippocampus is the brain area involved in short- and long-term memory as well as spatial navigation – an essential skill for taxi drivers. Enhancing this supports you in remembering names, numbers and nuances of conversation, while also helping you to navigate more easily.

As it is a complex task which involves a very wide brain network, learning a language can build cognitive reserve and provide a protective buffer against age-related decline. On top of the benefits to your brain, learning a new language can naturally expand your horizons and enrich your experiences in the world as it opens up new places and cultures.

WAYS TO ENGAGE YOUR LOVE OF LEARNING

- Ask interesting questions. Stay curious.
- Read a book.
- Learn a new language.
- Listen to a new podcast.
- Join a class, in person or online.
- Start a new hobby.
- Go to an event.

One of the consequences of biological ageing is that brain cells become less able to cope with cellular inflammation and free radicals. Just like your body, the brain becomes less malleable and resilient to stress as the connections between brain cells – also known as synapses – begin to erode. Because of the intricate architecture of your brain structure (86 billion neurons forming 100 trillion connections!), initially your brain can compensate by forming new connections through a process known as neurogenesis. Eventually, however, the reduction in BDNF (brain-derived neurotrophic factor) leads to loss of brain volume, which averages about 5 per cent per decade from the age of 40 onwards.

Which brings me to the story of Sr Bernadette of the Notre Dame order of nuns. When Sr Bernadette died from a heart attack at the age of 85, her brain, along with hundreds of others, was donated to scientific research as part of David Snowdon's *Ageing with Grace* project. He was studying the School Sisters of Notre Dame, a worldwide religious institution of Catholic sisters who lived almost identical lives in terms of lifestyle habits and daily schedules. Despite the similarities in their lifestyles, however, some of the nuns declined in terms of their memory and cognitive capacity, while others retained their capabilities for much longer. David Snowdon wanted to find out why.

Throughout their time in the order, the nuns subjected themselves to regular tests of brain function and memory. In addition, Snowdon examined the original essays written by the nuns decades earlier when they had entered the order as young novitiates. He was interested in the degree of grammatical complexity and idea density in the essays. As a result, he found that education and learning provided protective brain benefits; specifically, those nuns with low idea density decades earlier were far more likely to develop Alzheimer's dementia, while those who used rare words in their essays were 12 times less likely to do so.

Back to Sr Bernadette, whose brain showed evidence of extensive Alzheimer's disease when analysed. In addition, she turned out to have the ApoE4 gene, thought to confer a genetic predisposition to dementia. But despite these findings, Sr Bernadette had displayed no evidence of memory issues when alive, not even when she was tested at the age of 84, a year before her death. Not only that, but throughout her life she had consistently scored in the top 10 per cent on tests of brain function. Snowdon was puzzled. How was this possible?

Sr Bernadette had spent her life constantly challenging and stimulating her mind, from debates about matters of public interest to dozens of mental puzzles and quizzes. She was an avid reader with an insatiable curiosity for people and the world around her. Her commitment to lifelong learning had built extra brain capacity – sometimes termed cognitive reserve – that had buffered her brain function from the everyday effects of structural brain loss. As a result, despite developing Alzheimer's disease, quite remarkably she showed no symptoms of memory loss or mental decay prior to her death at the age of 85.[3]

Aside from keeping your memory in tip-top shape, learning new things can have so many benefits. Learning can make it easier to embrace change, broaden perspectives and build resilience. It can boost creativity, curiosity and critical thinking, while the sense of achievement from learning a new skill or hobby can be immense. As you learn, you broaden your mind and boost your self-confidence. A shared hobby or interest can provide the glue to connect and collaborate with others, thereby strengthening and supporting your social connections. But perhaps more than anything, learning new things can be fun, bringing more zest and excitement into your life. And there have never been so many ways to learn, from podcasts and online discussions to classes, courses and conferences.

It's never too late, either. Bill is thinking about going back to college as a (very) mature student. He recently read about someone in America who had completed their PhD aged 94.

'If he can do it, so can I,' Bill said.

Yes indeed. To learn is to live. Never stop learning and never stop growing – your future self really will thank you for it.

Commit to making memories

'Moments big as years' was poet John Keats' description of experiences that can be so powerful as to remain with you for all of your life. A feature of post-pandemic life has been an increased desire to invest in such experiences. After spending the best part of two years stuck in one place, many of us have a renewed interest in travelling to see different places and embrace new cultures. Many of us have also realised, after spending our locked-down days shopping online and splurging on various unnecessary 'pandemic purchases' that are now cluttering up our homes – think bread makers, expensive exercise equipment and unused musical instruments – that buying things is not the same as buying happiness.

Of course, you don't have to travel halfway across the world to have a memorable experience. A simple coffee break conversation with friends, a family event or weekend time in nature may all be equally emotionally resonant, fulfilling and memorable in their own way. Published research from the American Psychiatric Association has found that spending money on simple experiences, such as time with family or dinner with friends, is far more likely to boost your happiness and wellbeing than spending on 'stuff'. They have highlighted the wellbeing benefit of experiences in terms of strengthening relationships while creating opportunities to make meaning. Furthermore, reminiscing about these experiences can further enhance happiness and sense of self.[1]

Simply bringing more novel and varied experiences into your everyday routine can enhance happiness too. Research published in the journal *Nature Neuroscience* examined the association between diversity in daily experience and the degree of positivity of emotional states. Using GPS trackers over several months, they asked participants to report how positively or negatively they felt via 'in the moment' text messaging. They noted a strong positive connection between variability in experiences and strongly positive feelings. Using MRI brain scans, they directly correlated this emotional positivity with the degree of enhanced brain activity, finding a greater correlation in brain areas associated with the processing of novelty and reward (the hippocampus and the striatum).[2]

But the modern world values material things – always bigger, better and newer than what we already have – and 'purchasing happiness' seems to be an option. Turn on the TV, listen to the radio or scroll social media and you will be exposed to relentless advertising that either directly or subliminally links the product on offer with you feeling happier. Nowhere does this message sing more loudly than on Instagram and other social media platforms, where we are encouraged to 'buy this' or 'wear that' as status symbols of success and satisfaction. As a result, it is more difficult than ever to resist impulsive buying, with more temptations than ever just a click or two away on your mobile device.

Material purchases trigger feelings of novelty and stimulate the substantia nigra, the brain region that releases dopamine, a neurotransmitter that drives pleasure and reward. The instant gratification from the pleasurable release of dopamine, combined with the 'delayed pain' of paying later on the credit card, makes it incredibly easy to be lured into the honey trap of online purchases. But instant gratification fades quickly and rarely translates into longer-term happiness.

Occasionally it does, if the purchase supports positive experiences longer-term. Perhaps that new bike purchase will bring with it fitness, fun times and shared experiences with friends or family. However, for most purchases, the glitter generally fades quickly, perhaps not long after the wrapping paper is off. This is the catch: that momentary satisfaction from your new purchase may provide a very short-lived and transient effect on your wellbeing. This is the principle of hedonic adaptation at work – the inbuilt tendency for your happiness to revert towards its baseline level, irrespective of circumstances. Separate research involving groups of lottery winners and victims of life-changing accidents found that in both cases, after about a year of ups or significant downs, people generally reverted to their pre-situational level of happiness.[3]

Comparing ourselves with others can be the most natural thing in the world but comparing 'things' can seriously derail your happiness. You may find that you are always 'looking over your shoulder', ruminating about missing out on other potential purchases at a similar price (also known as the maximising effect) and negatively comparing your purchases to the perceived bigger or better purchases of other people. Negative comparison can trigger ingratitude, entitlement and envy, and the result may be that your own purchase quickly loses its sparkle. A reminder, perhaps, of *caveat emptor* – let the buyer beware; or perhaps more accurately, coveter beware – be careful what you wish for.

However, money can buy you happiness in the sense that it can provide peace of mind through financial security, protection in the event of emergencies and access to more choices, in addition to basic security in life. There are many material things you need: a roof over your head, transport, clean clothing, fresh food – the necessities. Money can also enable you to have enriching experiences. Positive experiences beat material purchases hands down when it comes to boosting subjective wellbeing and happiness; while any uplift in happiness from material purchases tends to be short-lived, experiences provide more substantial long-term wellbeing benefits. Investing in experiences can support your hobbies, interests, life goals and passions as well as connecting you with your sense of purpose. This can provide a deep well of fulfilment.

Positive experiences support feelings of gratitude in the moment and later as you reminisce on them. Of course, as we discovered in an earlier chapter, feeling grateful is a terrific way to reduce stress while boosting inner feelings of happiness and wellbeing. Investing in positive experiences can provide a lifetime of reflected happiness, memories and contentment. There is no expiration date on banked experiences; by contrast, they compound over time because of the inbuilt tendency to look back on your life through relatively 'rose-tinted' spectacles. Just think about some memorable experiences from your own life, such as precious time spent with family or friends.

How you choose to think about your experiences matters. One of the best ways to savour a past experience is to simply recall a positive experience in your mind. Think about the place and people you encountered, the sounds, smells, textures and physical sensations that you experienced. Think back to the emotions that you felt at the time. Let it all flow through you for a few moments. By doing this you aren't just reliving the experience – you are savouring it.

Savouring is defined as 'attending, appreciating, and enhancing positive experiences that occur in one's life'.[4] As a wellbeing tool, savouring can both bring you back to a positive experience and bring forward the associated positive emotions to enhance present-moment lived experience. This choice to consciously savour happy times can dissipate feelings of anxiety, providing an antidote to stress by lowering levels of stress hormones such as cortisol. As you better regulate your emotional responses to stress, you support emotional intelligence and enhanced resilience.

Travelling can really broaden the mind and create lasting memories. A simple change of scene for a day can do the trick, as can spending some time in health-enhancing environments in the natural world. Of course, experiences can challenge you to leave the security of your comfort zone and inspire you to embrace a new challenge or opportunity – something perhaps you've never done before. Running the New York Marathon back in 2007 was one such experience for me.

Sharing positive experiences with others creates mutual memories to last a lifetime. Think of a celebration with friends, a family holiday or another milestone. These experiences strengthen your sense of connection and support interpersonal relationships in many different ways. Sharing experiences and reminiscing about them builds emotional closeness, a sense of togetherness and a transcendent connection to something bigger than yourself. It serves as a reminder that you are part of the interconnected web of humanity.

A study was carried out in which participants were asked to list their top five lifetime material purchases and their top five lifetime experiential purchases (in other words, money spent on experiences) and then to write about their life's meaning. The researchers found that participants were twice as likely to include their experiential purchases rather than their material purchases when describing their life story. Why not try this exercise for yourself and see what matters most to you?[5]

Experiences expand and enhance your sense of self, informing who you are. Every experience forms part of the jigsaw of your life, another page in your autobiography. By embracing the depth and richness of your experiences, you are living life by the timeless advice of '*Mori memorias, non somnia*', meaning 'die with memories, not dreams'.

Positive experiences are a tremendous source of purpose and meaning. They can provide a treasure trove of timeless memories that may cost next to nothing apart from the gift of your time or energy. Some might require a little investment while others may be the price of 'a trip of a lifetime'. The science strongly suggests that investing in positive experiences is invaluable for your wellbeing. Ultimately only you can decide how to spend your time and resources, but before you make your next material purchase, perhaps ask yourself whether this is something you need or whether the funds could be spent on an experience. Even better, is there a meaningful experience you could plan that won't hurt your wallet or bank account? Instead of scrolling endlessly for another so-called bargain, call a friend or go for a walk in nature instead. Next month, when the buzz of instant gratification has long since passed, your future self will thank you for being so wise. Less dopamine and instant gratification perhaps, but more durable gold from sustainable happiness.

Find your purpose

Nature versus nurture is a long-standing debate about the relative influence on human beings of their innate biology (or 'nature') and the environmental conditions of their development (or 'nurture'). Nowadays, most experts acknowledge that nature and nurture both play a role in our psychological development, and they are intricately linked in many complicated ways. However, a third component is often overlooked: narrative. Your narrative is made up of the stories you tell yourself over and over again. These stories influence your values, inform your choices and shape your destiny in so many ways. They connect what we do to who we are and our sense of purpose. And while you can't change your genes or upbringing, you are always the author of your own life story.

I'm reminded of Margaret, who had worked her way up from the factory floor to become the human resources director in a global organisation headquartered in Dublin. When she came to me a number of years ago in my medical practice, she had been under a great deal of stress. A major restructuring within her company had meant that that she was being made redundant at 50 years old. Tears flowed as she reflected on her life and career. Her dad had died when she was still in primary school and opportunities for further education had been limited. Margaret had the added responsibility of being the eldest of five children and wanted to help out her financially stretched mother. As a result, she had taken a factory job straight after school. As the conversation continued, Margaret commented that she had never wanted to work in HR anyway – it was simply something she had fallen into.

'Then what did you want to do?' I probed gently.

'Oh, that's easy,' said Margaret. 'I was always fascinated by law. I wanted to fight injustice and defend those people unable to defend themselves.'

'So why don't you go back and study law now?' I asked.

Margaret looked at me as if I was mad.

'Sure, that would take at least five years. I'd have to go back to college, study for a law degree, then take more specialist exams after that. What's more, in five years' time, I will be 55 years old!'

My question to Margaret was 'What age will you be in five years' time if you don't go back and study law?'

Of course, as children, few of us know how we want to spend our lives. But as you grow up, with the benefit of life experience, you become wiser. And when you know more, you can do more and become more. Little by little, in aligning your passions to your strengths, you can serve the world in a way that allows you to be valued, whether by making a living or by making a difference in the lives of others.

Reconnecting with your purpose will likely improve your longer-term health as well. It supports a healthier heart, lowering risk of heart attack and stroke.[1] Purpose encourages you to become a more active participant in your own wellbeing and take full responsibility for your life. It strengthens your sense of self, makes you better able to embrace stress and enhances your capacity to gain new perspectives and to grow.

When asked how he created his masterpiece 'David', Michelangelo reputedly said that he simply started with a block of marble and gradually chipped away at everything that didn't belong, revealing the authentic essence of the sculpture hidden within. Many people find themselves similarly encased in a block, partly of their own making and partly as a result of the pervading beliefs and cultural norms of their environment. Sometimes, old insecurities or fears can keep you stuck right where you are. But we can choose to embrace that vulnerability, to leave the comfort zone and instead choose courage; the courage to face those fears of change and to simply take the first step.

Revealing your inner self requires a stripping away of old stories that no longer serve you. The result of connecting with your inner purpose is revealing a priceless masterpiece – your truest self.

In terms of the work you do, you have the capacity to change your inner story about it, irrespective of your work environment. Research from Yale University found that people have varying perspectives about their work, seeing it either as a job, a career or a calling. Regardless of job type – professor or plumber, doctor or delivery man, waiter or window cleaner – about a third of workers fell into each category.

For those people who see their work simply as a job, the emphasis is on the pay cheque and the work is done out of necessity. Their work may provide very little fulfilment for them, which can be a recipe for major work dissatisfaction, particularly if compensation is perceived as inadequate.

If you view your work as a career, you are more likely to be personally invested in the work and committed to succeeding as a result. The perceived rewards are external in nature – for example professional development, recognition and prestige. This can drive people for a long time, and they may spend years climbing a ladder of achievement, only to reach the summit and feel empty, devoid of purpose and meaning.

If you see your work as more of a calling, you probably love what you do, perhaps even to the extent that you would keep doing it for free if you could afford to. Because you see your work as being meaningful, having a higher purpose and making a positive contribution to the world, you are happy to work for the sake of the work itself. The real rewards are internal for you as you get to use your innate strengths. As you are more invested in this type of work, you will persist and persevere longer and be more likely to succeed as a result.[2]

Here's the key finding: workers who see their work as a calling or vocation have much higher job satisfaction[3] and overall life satisfaction[4] than people who simply see their job in terms of clocking in and out and collecting the pay cheque. Seeing your work as a calling depends not on your position or salary but simply on the degree of purpose and meaning you choose to find in your work. Living your why on a daily basis, at work and in life, is a reminder that you can make your own meaning by intuitively understanding that what you do matters, whether at a micro or macro level. Seeing your work as a calling takes courage.

Just as there are engineers and executives who see their work simply as a job, so there are street cleaners who see their work as a calling. Martin Luther King put it so well when he said, 'If a man is called to be a street sweeper, he should sweep streets even as Michelangelo painted, or Beethoven composed music or Shakespeare wrote poetry. He should sweep streets so well that all the hosts of heaven and earth will pause to say, "Here lived a great street sweeper who did his job well."'

One of the more helpful ways to reframe your mindset about work is to focus less on the monetary aspects of the job and more on ways in which you can use your strengths to serve and support others. Through this lens of service, a fireman is still someone who extinguishes fires but also someone who keeps communities safer, supporting community wellbeing. A schoolteacher is not just a teacher but a mentor and inspirational leader for the next generation of young people. A hospital janitor is not just a cleaner but someone who contributes to patient safety, helping to keep hospitals freer of infection, safeguarding health and lives. As you recraft and reorientate your job description towards service, you feel more fulfilled as you connect more closely to your why.

Of course, work is only one of the ways in which you may measure your life, with many other paths to purpose and a life of meaningful contribution. Make time to do more of what you love to do, follow your heart and find your flow. Master the art of fulfilment, which of course is unique for each person. Move away from who you are being based on status or possessions and towards an identity determined by inner core experiences and core values. Allow things to unfold more naturally with ease and synchronicity in alignment with your true nature.

As a human being (not human doing), it is so important to strip away all the superficiality of life to remind yourself what, deep down, you really, really want in life. Take some time to reflect on the purpose and meaning of your life, realigning your goals to your own values as opposed to the expectations of others. Use your strengths to express your talents and be of more service to others. Give time and energy through volunteering to build a better world. Choose to be part of something greater than yourself, connecting with people who share your values and make you feel valued and appreciated. Explore your spirituality by living out a personal act of faith.

The time has passed and today Margaret has fulfilled one of her lifelong dreams by going to university to study law. But you don't need to change careers or choose a different life path in order to find meaning in every day. There are simply so many ways that you can create a stronger sense of purpose in the ordinary day-to-day experiences of life. Awareness is the starting point for positive change, so open the door to this inner journey of self-discovery. Redefine what real purpose means for you and become crystal clear on what living your why might look like. Start today to reignite your purpose and experience more fulfilment. Your life is simply too short not to dream your dreams and live on purpose at your highest potential. Your future self will be glad you did.

Start a path to financial freedom

How do you rate your financial wellbeing right now? Are you on a solid footing or struggling to keep your head above water?

The financial crash of 2008 in Ireland brought with it a tsunami of misery. Many people experienced financial distress, with mortgages, careers and futures underwater. There were so many individuals who crossed my surgery door at that time with symptoms of severe stress, anxiety and fear of an increasingly uncertain future. This was when I really came to appreciate what a catastrophic impact financial distress can have on a person's overall subjective wellbeing.

The reality is that many people are struggling financially, caught up in a never-ending spiral of debts, crushed under the weight of financial commitments or consumed by a cycle of impulse buying. Whatever the circumstances, the bottom line is that many people feel highly stressed about money.

I am reminded of Adam, a young man of 28 who came to see me recently for a check-up. His partner was a stay-at-home mum to their two young children while he worked as a general operative in a multinational pharma company. With two young children, life had been busy for them, and he had been neglecting his own self-care and was (understandably) sleep deprived, sedentary and subdued. While Adam wasn't overtly depressed, he seemed stressed and it was evident to me that his well-being was low. I tried to home in on the underlying cause. There was no significant work-related stress, and he didn't drink to excess, gamble or struggle with addiction.

'How is your financial health?' I asked, well aware that many people are struggling right now due to the rising cost of living. Adam began to open up about the constant struggle to keep his head above water financially. He and his partner were renting a two-bedroom apartment and had been hoping to save for a mortgage, but this was proving impossible. Worse than that, he always seemed behind on his bills. His partner liked to shop online, and what had started out as an occasional purchase had turned into weekly, and sometimes daily, arrivals by courier van. Most of the purchases were small – matching outfits for their young daughters, beauty products and household furnishings – but they were adding up at such speed that Adam feared it was jeopardising their financial future.

My suggestion was a referral to MABS, the local Money, Advice and Budgeting Service, for support and practical advice on financial wellbeing. When I saw Adam again, he told me that he felt much better. Their time with MABS had proved very helpful. Adam's partner had admitted that her impulse buying was a way of coping with the stress of being home with two young children all day, and Adam realised he needed to be open about his financial concerns and discuss them with her instead of bottling them up. Now for the first time ever, they had a financial plan and were working together as a team, setting (and sticking to) a monthly budget.

Financial stress can have a very negative impact on your mental wellbeing. According to research by *Forbes*, experiencing financial stress means you become twice as likely to report overall poor health and four times more likely to complain of a range of health issues ranging from feeling fatigued, anxious and depressed to head-aches, migraines, digestive problems, sleep disturbance and raised blood pressure.[1] Which is why developing confidence and feelings of security around financial well-being is so important for your future self.

At a social occasion recently, I gravitated towards an older man who was sitting quietly at the kitchen table. After chatting with him a while, I learned that he had enjoyed a fascinating career in insurance. He told me about how he started out in working life many years earlier with his first job as postboy for a large insurance firm. Each day, his responsibility was to hand-deliver the mail to the various departments of the large London corporation, ending up at the door of the managing director.

'Over time I got to know this man, and gradually he took an interest in my own personal development,' he told me. 'He was a tremendous role model and over the years gave me plenty of great advice – but it was his financial advice that proved priceless.

'The first thing he told me was that knowledge is key. He said that I should keep a precise budget over a month or two so that I knew exactly where every penny was going. Secondly, he advised me to live on 70 per cent of what I earned. I was a young man with no dependents, so this was easy! Thirdly, he advised me to take 10 per cent and give it away to people less fortunate than me, through my local church, St. Vincent de Paul or the like. Such small contributions can make a big difference. And finally, he advised that I take the remaining 20 per cent and save it, either by putting it into a high-interest savings account or by paying into a pension, which I started in my twenties.

'I'm so glad I took his advice now. Of course, in the first few years I did without a few nice things, but I didn't starve. More importantly, it gave me the financial discipline to think twice before I bought things. I think it's much harder for young people nowadays, with all the pressure to keep up. But the fundamentals of financial security haven't changed one iota.'

Actions do speak louder than words and financial freedom starts with taking active steps to improve your financial circumstances. Do a review of your current spending patterns and saving habits. Accepting the reality of how things are right now, today, is the starting point to make positive changes.

Kakeibo (pronounced 'kah-keh-boh') is a Japanese practice that supports you to save more while spending less through more mindful financial choices. It offers a more nuanced approach to your finances, underscored by a Japanese philosophy of life which emphasises simplicity, harmony and sustainability.

The essence of kakeibo is the practice of carefully recording your financial income and expenses by hand in a journal. The term translates to 'household financial ledger', underscoring this somewhat 'old world' approach of keeping a ledger to track income and expenses. It is a process that builds awareness of why you spend what you spend. In a nutshell, it changes your relationship with your spending choices as you become more mindful about them.

There are four separate categories of spending in kakeibo. These are needs (living essentials, groceries, household bills, etc.), wants (eating out, gadgets, optional items of clothing, etc.), culture (arts, theatre, concerts, books, charity or other educational development) and finally, the unexpected (think emergency expenses such as car maintenance, medical, dental, plumber, etc.). You may have additional or different columns, which is absolutely fine. What matters is that you are using this written practice to record your spending in each of the different areas. By simplifying your budget, you can see the bigger picture. For example, is that new outfit a necessary 'must have' for work or is it simply a 'want to have' for the next night out?

The culture category is important as it recognises that you work to live as opposed to the other way round. Money is a vehicle to support a meaningful life well lived, rather than the end point in itself.

A key element of the kakeibo practice at the beginning and subsequently at regular (ideally weekly) intervals is reflection. By reflecting on questions that connect you with your values, they become front and centre in your financial decision-making and help reorient your finances towards living a more meaningful life. The questions are: 'How much money are you spending in each of the four areas? Did any of your spending surprise you? How much money do you have? Did you save what you planned to save? How can you maintain your progress, tweak your plans or make improvements next time?'

This process of regular reflection can help you take back control of your spending habits, boosting your confidence in your money management skills. If you find it difficult to keep to a budget, give it a try and see for yourself. It's accessible to everyone and, best of all, it's absolutely free. Kakeibo can support you to manage your money more mindfully and sustainably today, while prudently providing for a more financially secure future you.

Tom Corley is an American author and motivational speaker. Having studied hundreds of people over a five-year period, he has gained fascinating insights into the significant differences between financially wealthy and financially poor people in terms of their everyday habits. He shared some of his insights with me in conversation on my podcast *In the Doctor's Chair*.

Tom described how those people with what he calls 'rich habits' have cultivated a strong sense of passion and purpose as they live their 'why' on a daily basis. He documented a commitment to self-improvement, reading and lifelong learning, with 85 per cent of study participants reading at least two books a month. Focusing on staying healthy was a top priority for most, with three in four making time for regular exercise, valuing sustainable self-care strategies over other destructive health-depleting habits. They tended to foster strong supportive relationships while, where possible, avoiding toxic relationships. They had mentors who provided support and constructive criticism to continue their growth trajectory. They also minimised distractions and avoided procrastination.

Self-discipline in health, relationships and productivity compounds over the years to create a roadmap to a more prosperous future you. Tom's analogy is sowing seeds; just like habits, these eventually bear the fruit of good fortune or failure.

It was interesting to me just how much overlap there is between Tom's observed 'rich habits' and habits for achieving optimal health and wellbeing. In his words, 'authoring the circumstances of your life starts with self-awareness. If you want to be wealthy, healthy and happy, you need to have a positive mental attitude. Surround yourself with people who will support you and lift you emotionally when you are down. Cultivate the growth habit – investing time and energy daily as your evidence of commitment to excellence. Become clear on future you five, twenty years from now. Write it down and design a blueprint for future you.'

Benefits of financial wellbeing include managing a budget, having better control of your spending habits, reducing and paying off debt, learning the habit of saving and preparing for major life expenses – including buying your own home, planning for your future and preparing for retirement. Maybe you want to travel, pursue your dreams, invest in your hobbies or engage in self-development. Perhaps you want to make memories or simply sleep more soundly at night. Financial wellbeing is a step forward to provide more freedom to enable you to do those things that matter most. Which is why the best time to begin to improve your financial wellbeing is today. Take that first step, make a plan and simply start. Your future self will be glad you did.

Embrace yoga

How much do you know about the practice of yoga? Perhaps you are already a devotee, attending classes and practising regularly at home; perhaps you have never so much as attempted a downward dog or tree pose in your life. A gentle work-out through a range of different poses (also called asanas) that support whole-body balance, flexibility and strength, yoga is a valuable way to strengthen and support the spinal muscles, thereby helping to build a stronger, more resilient spine less prone to back or neck pain.

But it is the deeper mind–body connection from yoga that resonates most with me. Yoga practice is very grounding in that it keeps you centred, humble and honest. It can be physically demanding, but as the famous quote goes, 'Yoga is not about touching your toes; it's about what you learn on the way down.'

In essence, yoga is a group of physical, mental and spiritual practices focused on bringing harmony between mind and body. It can also build strength and flexibility while helping to better manage pain and stress. Dating back thousands of years, the word 'yoga' comes from the Sanskrit root '*yuj*' meaning 'root' or 'to unite'; as in, moving away from any sense of separateness and back towards an integrated wholeness of mind, body and spirit. With a mindful focus on the breath and attentive aware-ness of the self, practising yoga moves you away from the fight-or-flight stress response and facilitates a state of progressive relaxation.

In my practice I have recommended yoga for many years to support mental relaxation, core strength and flexibility, particularly to sufferers of back pain. Having dabbled in it myself several years ago, one of my current commitments to my own wellbeing has been to build a regular yoga practice into my week. I'm still very much a beginner, with lots of stops and starts, but the semblance of a longer-term habit is starting to emerge. Of course, it's all about awareness and being a beginner is no bad thing, as the 'beginner's mind' is known to be a place of openness, gratitude, compassion, non-attachment and humility. The last time I could touch my toes to my ears I was a baby, so there's plenty of room still to learn!

One of the main goals of a yoga practice is to find your edge, a place where your mind is still, your focus is on your breath, and you are stretching (but not over-whelming) yourself physically. One of the great paradoxes of yoga is that poses and movements that seem so disarm-ingly simple can prove to be so deceptively difficult!

Perhaps more importantly, the experience is restora-tive and highly relaxing. After a recent class I was surprised to find how chilled, energised and recharged I felt, which was in sharp contrast to how I had felt before at the end of a long and busy day at work. No one is immune from the microstresses that each day can bring to us all; those little things that you may not even have a real awareness of, but that subconsciously have an impact. Each microstress produces another small dose of stress hormones, and over time this has the potential to negatively impact your wellbeing in so many ways. This is why allowing your-self to regularly recharge from stress is so important. Yoga encourages and empowers you to become a more active participant in your own wellbeing and life journey. As written in the *Bhagavad Gita*, it is 'the journey of the self, through the self, to the self'.

Research published in the *International Journal of Yoga* has highlighted the multiple potential benefits from a regular yoga practice that go way beyond building strength and supporting posture, flexibility and balance.[1] Yoga has been found to help reduce feelings of stress, anxiety and depression, while supporting more restful sleep. It can help with chronic pain, recovery from addiction through chemical and emotional sobriety, and support heart health and healthier ageing.[2]

Yoga can have significant benefits for your mental wellbeing by fine-tuning the mind–body connection and lowering feelings of stress. As a complementary treatment for mood disorders such as depression and anxiety, yoga may have long-lasting benefits, and it may also have some benefits as an add-on treatment to support survivors of post-traumatic stress disorder (PTSD). Yoga may be considered an effective form of mind-body medicine as it focuses on integrating various elements of wellbeing (mind, body, emotion, spirit) in a way that improves wellbeing and combats stress.

But what about those of us who don't have significant mental health challenges? It turns out that investing in yoga might be one of the best things you can do to enhance your brain capacity, supporting a sharper, more highly attuned brain.

Yoga supports the growth of new brain cells (also known as neurogenesis) and the creation and strengthening of brain connections (also known as neuroplasticity), particularly in areas that support memory, awareness, attention, learning, language, rational thought, reasoning and decision-making. The result is an improvement in the brain's executive functioning capacity and sharpness. Think of it as being like a workout for the brain. This is supported by research involving brain scans which led to two key findings: firstly, those who do yoga have visible changes to the cerebral cortex, an area of the brain that deals with learning, memory and information processing; secondly, while these brain areas tend to shrink with age, older people who did yoga experienced less age-related shrinkage, supporting the connection between yoga and a sharper, more youthful brain.[3]

Of course, yoga benefits the body as well as the brain. It is classified as a form of complementary and alternative medicine by the American National Institutes of Health, and research suggests that yoga can help lower blood pressure in those with diagnosed hypertension. This is possibly due to an effect on baroreceptor sensitivity, helping to balance blood pressure. Yoga is also considered a helpful intervention to support cardiac rehabilitation after a cardiac event and, perhaps more importantly, for heart disease prevention.

As a form of exercise and movement, yoga can produce significant mood-boosting benefits by reducing stress hormones such as cortisol while raising levels of positivity neurochemicals such as serotonin, dopamine, noradrenaline and endorphins. It can also trigger the release of gamma-aminobutyric acid (GABA) from the thalamus in the brain. GABA puts the brakes on feelings of anxiety, producing feelings of calm.[4]

The associated slow movements and deeper, more mindful breathing of yoga practice dampen brain activity in the brain's emotional areas, known as the limbic system. This reduces emotional reactivity and plugs you into the pause-and-plan parasympathetic nervous system. This is a place of less anxiety and greater calm, less anger and greater peace, less distraction and greater presence. It builds a sense of openness, optimism and emotional equanimity that can boost your everyday energy and vitality.

Mindfulness refers to paying attention to what you are experiencing in the present moment, on purpose and without judging yourself. Overall, a regular yoga practice can support more mindful living, helping you to be more present in other areas of your life. This includes a more positive relationship with food in general. More mindful eating may result from an increased mind–body connection as your awareness of hunger cues and feelings of fullness improves. Research has found that yoga can positively impact body mass index and support a healthier weight through a more positive relationship with food.[5]

Spiritually, yoga can provide a foundation for inner peace and contentment by creating the conditions for calm presence. Yoga is one of the ways to move back towards what I call 'true self' – a place of heightened present-moment awareness. A place that acknowledges, but lets go of, the past. A place that appreciates the potential power that exists in the present moment and anticipates the 'next steps' with openness and optimism. Grounded in gratitude and connection to self, others and your higher power, true yoga embraces the experience of unity, of wholeness, of interconnectedness. As such, the self becomes submerged into a new reality, dissolved into an invisible oneness. There is no longer 'in here' in your subjective experience and 'out there' in the world. This is the mindset of yoga, and you can practise this mindset even if you never join a class or practise the asanas.

Hopefully reading this chapter may inspire you to discover whether yoga is something that might be for you. If it does, here is some advice to guide you on your path of exploration.

Get the go-ahead

Before starting, take full responsibility for your wellbeing by ensuring that a yoga practice is safe for you, particularly if you have significant spinal issues in your neck or back. Consult your doctor of physiotherapist if needed.

Practise self-acceptance

Yoga starts on the inside with complete acceptance of your current reality in the present moment. It lets go of self-criticism that you can't touch your toes or that your back is stiff and self-judgement that you are too old, fat, thin or whatever negative message your inner critic is sending you right now. Instead, you appreciate the gift of your body right now and start with a spirit of mindful self-acceptance.

Start slowly

Yoga is slow, steady and mindful. There are many different poses possible, both on and off the mat. Chair yoga is another option for people with significant spinal or mobility issues. Move gently and mindfully through the various poses and keep within the limits of what's possible for your body. Focus on a healthy stretch, never going beyond that to the point of pain or discomfort.

Be fully present

Release into each pose fully and completely as you bring your present moment awareness to the breath and your body. Become aware of sensations as they arise and let go of thoughts that emerge as you stay present and relaxed in your posture and breath.

Never stop starting

It's never too late to start. Commit to a regular practice – even a few minutes a few times a week will compound, creating significant benefits over time.

THREE YOGA POSES YOU CAN DO WITHOUT A MAT

Mountain pose

Stand with your feet together, heels slightly apart. Press into all four corners of your feet. Feel the muscles in your legs engage.

Roll your shoulders up and release them back and down. Keep your neck nice and long.

Take a few deep breaths.

Forward fold

As you inhale, take your arms out to the sides and up over your head.

On your exhale, release your arms down in front of your body as you fold your torso over your legs. Keep a slight bend in your knees.

Gently place your hands on your shins. This lengthens your spine and your hamstrings.

As you take a few deep breaths and begin to relax into the pose, you can straighten your legs out as far as feels good.

Plank pose

From a forward fold position, put your hands flat on the floor, bending your knees as much as necessary to do so. Step back one leg at a time, until you're in a high plank.

Press into your hands, keeping your legs parallel and engaged. Pull your bellybutton toward your spine.

Take a few deep breaths here, working your core and your arms.

Overall, yoga can provide a range of benefits that positively impact your physical, mental, emotional and spiritual wellbeing. It offers a pathway from energy depletion to energy enhancement, from resistance to flow and from stress to serenity. Think more clearly in the present moment, feel more balanced and positive and act more in alignment with your values.

Finally, yoga encourages and empowers you to become a more active participant in your own wellbeing and life journey. By taking more ownership of your health journey, each yoga practice becomes a step forward into enhanced wellbeing, one breath and mindful movement at a time.

Nurture your spiritual side

Do you engage in prayer, or reflect on the purpose and meaning of life events? Do you spend time in stillness or silence? Are you tolerant and considerate of the views of others, even when they are different from your own? Are your choices and decisions guided by your values? Do you make time for meditation? In other words, do you take time to nurture your spiritual side?

American academic and author Brené Brown defines spirituality as 'recognising and celebrating that we are all inextricably connected to each other by a power greater than all of us, and that our connection to that power and to one another is grounded in love and compassion'.[1]

It is a bridge between you and a higher power or wider universe; a bridge that allows you to travel into and discover a deeper purpose and sense of meaning; to find comfort, guidance and inner peace in times of struggle.

Perhaps you are wondering why I have chosen to include a chapter on spirituality in this book, given that I am a medical doctor who, by definition, has a grounding in science. For many, the paradigm of duality requires a clear separation between the two, with evidence-based science completely disconnected from the 'woo-woo' world of spirituality. However, I have personally treated patients for whom faith has facilitated recovery from illness. It has enabled many others to find comfort, fostering healing and providing them with a beacon of hope and light as they find their way back from addiction and other health problems.

To quote Albert Einstein, 'Everyone who is seriously involved in the pursuit of science becomes convinced that a spirit is manifest in the laws of the Universe – a spirit vastly superior to that of man, and one in the face of which we with our modest powers must feel humble.' As I see it, you have a choice: to see science and spirituality as separate entities or as synergistic elements of a larger, interconnected wholeness. You can live purely through the lens of science with its 'show me the evidence' objectivity, disregarding subjective spiritual experience. On the other hand, you may be a serious spirituality seeker and choose to ignore the objectivity of scientific facts.

As a doctor I choose to lean into the subjective experience of spirituality with a scientific mind. By appreciating that we are all interconnected and underpinned by a universal consciousness, we can choose both. This is a journey of self-discovery from separateness to wholeness, and from divisive dualism to a more inclusive unity; being comfortable in not knowing all the answers and accepting that some answers are simply unknowable.

While many people express their spirituality through personal acts of religious faith, others do so by being present in nature, meditating, spending time in stillness or silence, or even by attending music or sporting events. Spirituality can also lead to discovery and self-realisation through the exploration and expression of your deeply held values.

Research involving thousands of people across cultures from India to China and the USA, with beliefs ranging from secular to religious, indicates that there are five separate elements to spirituality.[2] These five elements are: the 'golden rule' (to love your neighbour as yourself), a sense of 'oneness' or interconnection, altruism, living in accordance with your values (a moral code) and a sense of sacred transcendence.

THE FIVE ELEMENTS OF SPIRITUALITY: GOALS

G: Golden Rule

O: Oneness

A: Altruism

L: Lived values

S: Sacredness

Research from Yale University has found evidence that when study participants recall a personal experience in vivid detail, the brain changes seen on fMRI mimic the actual experience itself. This finding forms the basis for groundbreaking research by Dr Lisa Miller on the neuroscience of spirituality, described in her book *The Awakened Brain: The Psychology of Spirituality*. Her study participants were asked to recall three separate experiences they had encountered – one stressful, one relaxing and one spiritual. They were encouraged to give detailed descriptions of these experiences, including the context and circumstances, as well as the granular details of their experience. About half of the spiritual experiences involved prayer or a religious service including a feeling of unity, while most of the remainder involved time spent in nature. A few experiences involved playing music or participating at a sporting event. Universally, the participants described experiencing a stronger sense of self with sharpening of the senses during these experiences. Their heart rates increased with a significant reduction in negative ruminating thoughts noted. They felt more alive, with more vitality and a strong emotional sense of peace, awe, clarity, openness and a profound sense of connection to and love for their higher power, other people or their environment. They also described moments of insight and clarity into unresolved issues in their life. This was all underpinned by a specific sense of meaning to the experience: a dissolving of boundaries, a unity or overwhelming connection resulting in an experience of oneness.

Two weeks later, the participants returned for part two of the investigation. This time they listened to their previous stories being replayed while they were physically ensconced in the fMRI scanner. The biological, physiological and neurological brain changes detected during the recall of the spiritual stories were significant and pretty much identical irrespective of their context (whether the experience was based in religion, nature, music or something else).

Firstly, there was a quieting of part of the brain known as the default mode network (DMN), an area involved with replaying ruminative, anxious and negative thoughts that take you away from present-moment awareness. Turning down this brain area through the experience of spirituality facilitates the 'small self' effect, whereby the ego dissolves as you become more open and attuned to a more expansive worldview.

Secondly, there was a change in the brain's attentional network, with this filtering system for brain inputs changing in a manner that improved the perception of information outside the normal bandwidth of experience. This shift can spark new perceptions, new perspectives and potential new clarity and creative insights.

Thirdly, there was heightened activity in brain areas dealing with relational connectedness and the experience of positive emotions, including love and bliss. And finally, there was a dampening of activity in the parietal lobe, which plays an important role in the perception of self and separateness. As this decreases, there is a perceived softening of boundaries between self and others, leading to an expanded sense of self and, beyond that, to a sense of transcendent oneness.[3]

The cortex is part of the brain where emotional stimuli are processed, and it is involved with mood, planning and reasoning. Research has found a correlation between cortical brain thickness and protection from depression in the presence of certain spiritual traits, including altruism and living by the golden rule. This might be due to the focus on connection with others rather than disconnection and self-centred isolation.[4]

Religion tends, for the most part, to encourage moderation and a lower-stress, healthier lifestyle. As a result, people with religious beliefs tend to be happier, better connected to their families and more satisfied with life overall. Through a sense of community, relationships can be strengthened by the significant social support that involvement in religious activity brings. Separately, improving your spiritual wellbeing may help you feel better physically, psychologically and emotionally. Spirituality can provide peace of mind, inner security and serenity. It may offer a buffer against the negative impact of other life stressors, including illness or bereavement, providing some protection against depression and a reduced risk of developing addiction.[5]

The sense of forgiveness and compassion for others that spirituality cultivates can build coping skills and support resilience. It promotes more positive engagement and relationships with self, with others and with your environment. Spirituality also supports self-acceptance; accepting yourself for who you really are, including your imperfections and shortcomings, while taking 100 per cent responsibility for your own life.

As a spiritual practice, meditation has been part of Sanskrit Indian philosophy and many structured religions for centuries. In recent times, it has been appreciated for its ability to calm the mind, bringing more presence and awareness to everyday experiences. Structural changes to the brain (known as neuroplasticity) have been documented in long-term meditators, who become more receptive to positive emotions such as enthusiasm and happiness, as part of the brain's 'happiness centre' in the left prefrontal cortex grows larger. In fact, as little as 11 hours of cumulative meditative practice, equating to just 10 minutes a day for three months, can lead to brain changes that quiet the amygdala, lower stress and boost self-awareness.

Meditation can increase heart rate variability, or HRV, a measure of overall balance in your nervous system associated with improved heart health. Regular meditation can support sleep and immune health, lower blood pressure and reduce feelings of anxiety, fatigue and chronic pain. An increase in grey matter in the brain can improve memory. It can also enhance impulse control and improve a person's relationship with themselves and others.

Meditation builds awareness of your own thoughts, emotions and interactions with others. It supports a stronger sense of self, a more positive self-image, and higher levels of self-confidence and self-esteem. It also builds emotional agility, reducing negative emotions while improving positive mood states. As a mindful practice, meditation changes brain waves from predominantly beta (associated with the busyness of the merry-go-mind) to more alpha wave activity, which is associated with deep relaxation and a journey to inner stillness. As you grow in awareness through inner knowing, you become more accepting and willing to take responsibility for things as they truly are. This provides a pathway to stillness and a deeper sense of being.

As a circuit breaker on stress, meditation supports a healthier, more resilient mind, leading to more restful presence and inner peace. It recharges the mind by upregulating activity in the hippocampus and prefrontal cortex while reducing activity in the amygdala. It increases self-control and self-regulation, making you feel less reactive and more responsive, less stressed and irritable, while cultivating a sense of calm and peace.

As a spiritual practice, meditation may lead to experiences of higher consciousness, intuitive wisdom and a sense of oneness with the universe. Spirituality is part of your nature – a hardwired trait that is part of your unique human potential. Approximately one-third of your spirituality is innate, while two-thirds is influenced by your family upbringing, environments, and lived experiences.[6] While you can't change your genes, you can choose how to engage with your environments and the world around you. Your spiritual wellbeing is an intensely personal experience, involving beliefs and values that provide purpose and meaning in your life. What works best for you may not work as well – or indeed, at all – for someone else. Be willing to experiment a little and see what fits you best.

WAYS TO STRENGTHEN AND SUPPORT YOUR SPIRITUAL WELLBEING

- Connect with a power greater than yourself
- Live out a personal act of faith
- Pray – alone or at a religious service
- Gift yourself some time in solitude
- Engage with music, literature or the arts
- Spend time in nature
- Meditate
- Recite mantras and affirmations
- Create a mandala (a sacred circle in Sanskrit) as a tool to assist with healing
- Volunteer or contribute to your community
- Read inspirational books
- Listen to inspirational podcasts
- Practise self-acceptance
- Live your values
- Build a sense of hope
- Keep a journal of little things that provide you with a sense of spirituality and transcendence (e.g., a beautiful sunset, inspiring words, witnessing an act of kindness)

Since mind, emotion, body and spirit are interconnected, spiritual wellbeing can strengthen these other elements, providing a sense of balance and harmony in life. The emotional comfort and strength gained from spirituality can enhance your self-esteem, boost confidence and contribute to healing. Spirituality can help combat feelings of helplessness, foster hope and deeper purpose, and instil the knowledge that who you are ultimately matters. It can cultivate gratitude and more positive feelings such as awe, fulfilment and inspiration, leading to a stronger sense of inner peace, security and serenity.

Think yourself younger

Imagine your only concept of age was based on how old you feel right now as you read this. What age is that, by the way? Is the number younger or older than your actual age?

It turns out that the age you believe and feel you are can make a big difference when it comes to your longevity, adding up to an extra seven years. Research published in 2002 in the *Journal of Personality and Social Psychology* involving hundreds of individuals aged 50 and older who participated in a community-based survey found that those people with a more positive attitude to ageing lived longer.[1] Specifically, it found that older individuals with the most positive self-perceptions of ageing lived on average 7.5 years longer than those with the most negative views. What proved fascinating was that this potential impact of mindset on ageing was independent of other variables including age itself, gender, socioeconomic status, serum cholesterol and blood pressure. These findings have since been replicated in many other countries from Germany to China and now form a key part of the World Health Organization's campaign for healthier ageing.

The precise mechanism by which a positive view of ageing impacts lifespan remains elusive. Perhaps people with a more positive view of ageing have a higher 'health IQ', are more likely to value their health, engage in more health-enhancing habits such as exercise, avail themselves of appropriate medical check-ups and take better care of themselves overall. Perhaps they have more of what the Japanese call *ikigai*, or inner purpose, with a more compelling reason to get up in the morning, whether by supporting others or making a meaningful contribution. Perhaps they deal better with stress or are grittier and more resilient, with a stronger 'will to live'.

This impact of mindset on ageing may reflect all of the above as well as other still unidentified factors. Whatever the underlying mechanisms, one thing is certain: a positive view of ageing is good for your long-term health and wellbeing!

Which brings me to Paddy, someone I had known for more than 25 years as a patient. While he lived within walking distance of my practice, he was someone I saw more often out and about in the neighbourhood than in my consulting room. Medically, he would be categorised as a fairly infrequent attender.

But it's a relatively recent interaction that I remember best. Paddy had attended for a routine check-up. As he sat opposite me, I was taken by the freshness of his appearance. He looked fit and strong in his leather jacket, jeans and Nike trainers.

'What age are you now, Paddy?' I asked as I looked over the medical record on my computer screen.

'Eighty-five,' Paddy answered.

'But what age do you feel?' I probed; the answer to this question can reveal much about mindset. 'I don't often see someone your age wearing such fashionable clothes,' I remarked.

'Oh, I've always believed in dressing much younger than I am,' he laughed. 'Sure age is all in your head. Truth told, I don't feel a day over sixty.'

While none of us can turn back the clock, Paddy's sentiment and physical demeanour got me thinking about the very real impact, both positive and negative, that mindset can have on your wellbeing and even the way in which you age. While Paddy was 85 based on his date of birth, he certainly didn't look, act or feel that age. What's fascinating about the term 'old age' is that there is no blood test or biological marker that a doctor can use to say, 'A*ha*, now we know what's wrong – you're old.' It's much more nuanced than that, which is why your beliefs about ageing and the actions that align with those beliefs can make such a difference to how you feel.

Imagine you are invited to a week-long retreat with several old friends. You are all going to spend time together in a lovely resort where you will roll back the years and reminisce on life many years earlier. You agree to undergo a variety of tests at the beginning and conclusion of your time together, including measures of ageing such as eyesight, grip strength and flexibility.

This is precisely what Harvard Professor Ellen Langer asked study participants to do in 1979 with her ground-breaking 'counterclockwise experiment', described in detail in the book *Higher Stages of Human Development.*[2] This experiment involved a group of eight men, all aged 75, who were invited to spend a week together at a resort. Their only instruction prior to arrival was to bring no books, magazines or material dated later than 1959 – 20 years earlier.

The men were told that during their time together they would be reflecting and reminiscing on what their lives had been like in 1959, when the participants were 55 years old.

They were also told that this experience would be beneficial to them. The location of the retreat and layout of the living quarters were intentionally designed to simulate the year 1959. All the newspapers, television programmes and movies available were from that time. All the kitchen and household appliances were also from 1959. Of note, all of the mirrors in the resort were removed.

Unknown to any of the participants, there was a second group of eight men who had also been invited to the resort. Described by Langer as the 'time capsule' group, their instructions differed in one key respect. Rather than simply remembering and reminiscing about life back in 1959, they were going to live out the week as if it were 1959 again. As such, the members of this 'time capsule' group were encouraged to speak in the present tense about 1959. They listened to songs by Perry Como and Jack Benny on a 1950s radio. Each day they took part in group conversations whereby current affairs and newsworthy events of that time – such as the Colts winning the National Football League, and Castro becoming prime minister of Cuba – were discussed as if they were actually happening contemporaneously. While the control group also discussed these events, for them it was simply through the lens of recollecting the past.

Before the retreat started, and again at its conclusion, all men were measured on various mental and physical parameters generally expected to disimprove and decline with age. These included physical strength, posture, perception, eyesight, cognition and short-term memory.

What the results revealed was remarkable and significant. After the retreat, many of the men in the 'time capsule' group had gained significant improvements in terms of hearing, hand grip strength, blood pressure, posture, flexibility and appetite. They were experiencing fewer aches and pains with improved overall subjective wellbeing. Memory and eyesight had also improved on average by about 10 per cent. While the men in the control group also documented measurable improvements, these weren't detected to the same degree as in the 'time capsule' group.

Perhaps most remarkably of all, the men looked younger. Photographs of each participant, taken before and after the retreat and independently assessed, found that men looked on average three years younger after just one week of 'thinking' themselves younger.

Dr Langer's own conclusion was that the interrelationship between mind and body is complex and powerful. Thinking yourself younger by going 'back in time' seemed to encourage the body to follow suit.

Research has also shown that subliminal exposure to positive words related to ageing may have a lasting positive impact, both in terms of physical functioning (walking speed, balance and ability to get into and out of a chair) and perceptions of ageing.[3] This highlights that the language you hear and use in relation to ageing can influence your wellbeing and may impact how you age – for better or for worse.

The world's longest study of ageing has been running since 1958 and continues to this day. Known as the Baltimore Longitudinal Study of Ageing, it carries out a detailed assessment of each study participant every two years. Dr Becca R. Levy, a leading researcher in the fields of social gerontology and psychology of ageing, has looked at the data and found that those with more positive age beliefs at the outset had 30 per cent better scores of memory function when older, an effect more powerful than that of degree of education, age or physical health.[4] Furthermore, she found that those with negative age beliefs were more prone to dementia. Specifically, the memory centres of their brains (hippocampi) shrank far more quickly, with an increased tendency to develop brain plaques signifying changes caused by dementia.

There is growing recognition of the close interrelationship between your mindset about ageing and health. A research study involving more than 14,000 patients aged over 50 found that a more positive attitude to ageing was associated with more purpose and optimism, with less loneliness or depression. Those with a more positive view of ageing had fewer chronic conditions such as heart disease and diabetes and better overall cognitive functioning. Furthermore, those people who reported the highest satisfaction with ageing had a massive 43 per cent lower risk of mortality from any cause during the study period. Separate research has also found that having a positive belief about ageing may support a faster and more complete recovery from illness or injury.[5]

Back to Dr Ellen Langer who, along with co-author Alia Crum, also carried out the 'chambermaid experiment'. This experiment involved an analysis of the exercise habits of 84 hotel maids, none of whom were taking any exercise of significance. Half of them were told that their daily work, such as making beds and cleaning bathrooms, was in fact exercise, just as if they had been working out at the gym. The other group of maids was given no such information.

Over a four-week follow-up period, and despite no change in exercise or eating habits from baseline, the 'my job is exercise' group lost weight, lowered their blood pressure and even reduced their blood cholesterol levels. The only difference between the two groups was the varying mindset and how that expected effect from exercise translated into tangible health gains. When it comes to your beliefs about your actions, the effect you expect may well be the effect you get.[6]

Of course, an obvious question to consider is whether your positive view of ageing reflects the fact that you are healthier to start with, as opposed to the positive attitude itself improving your health. Research strongly suggests the latter – that people are healthier primarily because of their positive ageing attitude, and not the other way around.[7][8]

So, if you're interested in developing a more positive mindset about ageing, start with awareness. Become more aware of your current attitudes and beliefs about ageing and older people. Are you enabling positive thoughts and beliefs, or reinforcing negative stereotypes, albeit subconsciously? Can you begin to see things differently, that your age is only a number? Can you bring more positive words for ageing into your everyday choices and language? Choosing to associate ageing with more positive words such as wisdom, creativity and vitality can make all the difference. Awareness is the starting point for meaningful positive change. It makes you more mindful of the people and places that pigeonhole older people.

Once you have cultivated awareness, you can choose to take action. Action means you choose to spend more time in environments and with people that celebrate ageing. To build more intergenerational social connections through hobbies, gatherings or community activities such as volunteering. Can you commit to valuing lifelong learning, while fostering a renewed sense of purpose? Can you embrace the belief that age is a wonderful asset to support you, as opposed to a hindrance to your hopes and dreams? Can you choose to not just look back on the past with rose-tinted spectacles, but forward too, with the rosiest spectacles you can imagine, gifting you a more optimistic view of ageing? An attitude of positivity, grounded in wisdom, can become a catalyst for a healthier future. A mindset that your future, older and wiser self will surely thank you for.

Visualise your future self

The Chinese bamboo tree grows in the Szechuan district of China. Also known as the 'lucky bamboo tree', there is a great deal of symbolism attached to it. It grows tall, strong and upright, symbolising great physical health, while its flexibility represents a resilient mind. It has a hollow centre, representing an open, unprejudiced heart full of compassion, empathy and optimism. In India the Chinese bamboo tree is a symbol of friendship, while in China it represents longevity. In feng shui, the Chinese bamboo tree is believed to bring positive energy to the home and to establish the proper balance between the natural elements of fire, earth, metal, wind and water.

From a health and wellbeing perspective, it also represents balance between the elements of mind, body, emotion, spirit and relationships.

Imagine planting a Chinese bamboo tree seed in a sunny aspect of your garden. You diligently feed, water and cultivate the soil around it each and every day for an entire year. Your hard work bears no visible result, but you don't give up. Instead, you persist in feeding, watering and cultivating the soil around the seed each day for four long years – which equates to 1,461 days. After four years, a small shoot appears, but aside from that there is no visible return for your efforts. Although your patience is beginning to fade, still you continue to nurture the seed. Then one day in year five, the Chinese bamboo tree breaks through the ground and begins to grow vigorously, reaching 27 metres tall in just five weeks! But did it really take just five weeks, or was it in fact five years?

For the first four years the Chinese bamboo seed was hard at work developing a complex, extensive root system to support its later upward growth. The growth was there all along – it was just hidden beneath the ground. The thing is, if on any of those days you hadn't taken the time to feed or water the seed, then the Chinese bamboo seed might have died in the ground and you would never have seen the fruits of your labours.

The seed of the Chinese bamboo tree represents possibility, the untapped potential of future you. The possibility that you can still your mind, silence your inner critic and support yourself to make the regular small investments in your wellbeing that future you will thank you for. These very same principles of nurturing the Chinese bamboo seed are applicable in your own life as well. While you may invest considerable time and effort to nurture your growth and improve your health, outward evidence of change can be slow, perhaps without any tangible results for weeks, months or even years. But with patience and persistence, your daily investments of time and effort will pay off.

The parable of the Chinese bamboo tree provides a reminder neither to shortchange your future self nor to allow others to write you off along the way in life. It highlights the key ingredients to successful long-term positive change: aligning vision to consistent action.

Visualisation is the process of forming a picture of something in your mind, seeing it through the lens of your imagination or very powerful subconscious mind. It can be a helpful technique to imagine your future self, to become clear on your goals and to better embrace stress. As Muhammad Ali once said, 'If my mind can conceive it and my heart can believe it, then I can achieve it.'

Before you visualise future you, it's important to create the right state of mind and get into the mood for visualisation. A short walk in nature is a wonderful way to boost creativity, while a mindful breathing exercise, written affirmation or guided meditation are other ways to ground you in presence. Simply sitting quietly in stillness can do the trick too. Once you have grounded yourself, close your eyes and picture your future self – in five, ten or fifteen years from now. Imagine that this future self travels to a beautiful destination. Not only can you see the wonderful vista, but you can smell, hear, feel and even taste this experience. Include as much sensory detail as possible – the sun on your skin, the smell of salt air or the trees around you, the sound of waves or running water. Now begin to visualise your future health. Perhaps your muscles feel strong beneath your skin, your eyesight is still clear and sharp and you are dancing or swimming without pain or fatigue. Finally, picture your relationships and self-development in the same multisensory way.

Writing a letter to your future self might, on the face of it, seem like an unusual request, perhaps akin to sending yourself a birthday card. However, this letter can become a compass to clarify your current position in life as well as signposting your future direction. It provides an opportunity to reinforce your strengths, restate your values, reimagine your goals (through activation of the reticular activation system in the brain), recognise those relationships that matter, reconnect to your purpose and reinforce feelings of appreciation through expressing gratitude. It creates a roadmap built on realistic optimism – the belief that things can get better because of your efforts and desire to do something about it. This draws you forward, day by day, towards that predesigned future version of you. Crystallise these ideas today by committing them to paper and you will essentially gift yourself a manifesto of sorts that future you can live by.

Start this letter-writing exercise by looking back to see how much you have grown and changed over the past five years. This allows you to create separation and space in your mind between your past and present selves. You can appreciate the differences in your relationships, outlook, perspective and worldview and gain valuable insights into who you are today, relative to where you were five years ago. Recognise the many differences between the person you were then and the person you are now, emotionally, mentally, spiritually and physically. This way, you can reframe the stories you tell yourself about your past, present and, more importantly, your future. The past is gone, while the present will soon be consigned to the past as well.

Looking back as an evaluation exercise can inform how you move forward into the future. How has this time been for you? How has your physical health been? How about your mental health and emotional wellbeing?

What about your relationships? Who are the people that have supported you or stressed you? With the benefit of hindsight, who would you have liked to have spent less or more time with? How did you celebrate the good times? How have you changed or grown over the past five years? What advice would you give yourself about the challenges you faced? What lessons have you learned? What might you have done differently with the benefit of hindsight?

Stepping outside of yourself to shine a light dispassionately on your life in this manner is the starting point to inform how you move forward through the lens of self-awareness. By seeing clearly the difference between your past and current self, you make it easier to envision your future self.

Having done this 'lookback exercise', you are now ready to write the letter that you are going to read five years from now. Think of it as being like the Chinese bamboo seed you are choosing to plant in your life today. Ultimately this exercise helps to give you back control over what matters most. Firstly, by reevaluating, and subsequently reorganising your life to move towards that more optimistic future version of you.

Imagine that five years from now, everything you have worked towards turns out for the best and you have become your best possible self. Think about the areas of life that matter most to you and the positive changes you'd like to see happen. As you think ahead, stay authentic and keep your plans real. Remember it's *your* best future self, not what you believe others or indeed society expects from you.

Start on the inside. Who do you want to be in five years' time, and why? What kind of life will you be living? What are the values that will guide you? What are the strengths that you will use? Next, think of the health habits you would like to build, the self-development you'd like to undergo, the books you'd like to read, the languages you'd like to learn. What about your career achievements and accomplishments? What are the hobbies you would like to learn and places you'd like to visit?

Who will you be living with? What about your family – which relationships will you prioritise and why? Who are the new friends you hope to make? How might this happen? What is the best family and social life you can imagine? What would stronger, more rewarding relationships look like for you? What impact are you having on others and on the world? How do others see you?

Be as specific as possible. What might be different compared to now? How does future you deal with challenges? How do you describe yourself? What do you look like, dress like? What habits – health and otherwise – does future you have that you currently have? What habits has future you cultivated that you don't have yet?

Wouldn't bringing all of this to fruition be exciting for you? Describe how will it feel when all these things come to pass. Be as specific and detailed as possible as you visualise this future you with insights into the connection between your everyday experiences and your future dreams.

Now it's time to start writing. Get it all down on paper over the next 15 minutes. Don't worry about spelling or grammar. This is a time to look forward, to be open and creative as you focus on your future potential as opposed to present problems or past experiences.

Having written your first draft, put it away for a day or two, or sleep on it at the very least, before returning to it with fresh eyes. Now it's time to redraft your letter to your best possible future self – to create version 2.0. Are there things you'd like to add in or take out? Having rewritten or edited your future self letter, read it out loud to yourself. How does it feel to read this?

Now ask yourself these important questions. Compared with this future version of you, how are you doing today? What are your gaps (we all have them!)? By this I mean the gap between who you are today and future you, the person whom you are capable of becoming? What are your gaps in terms of your health, goals, values and relationships? More importantly, how can you start to close those gaps? What's the smallest step you can take today that will provide you with evidence that you are moving in the direction of the person you wish to become?

Put the letter into an envelope, seal it and put it away somewhere safe to be opened at a designated future date. Five years is a long time – not too long, but long enough to make significant investments into future you.

Another way of imagining your future self is to get creative and draw it. Drawing is an active process that requires your brain to process information in multiple ways simultaneously that encode learning and deepen the impact. Firstly, there is the kinaesthetic memory from the pencil or pen physically connecting with paper through the act of drawing. Secondly there is the visual memory from what is drawn, and thirdly the semantic memories created through the meaning of what is drawn. This multilayered impact on memory through drawing your best possible future self can have a powerful impact, maybe even more so than visualisation or writing.[1] Perhaps a picture does indeed tell a thousand words.

Remember you don't need to be Picasso to partake in this exercise; you just need to be willing to take some crayons or colouring pencils and draw future you on a sheet of paper. Imagine that this drawing represents the landscape of your life. You are free to put in anything and everything that you believe represents future you. Suspend any ideas of not being 'good' at drawing – that doesn't matter one iota. What does matter is your willingness to express your dreams and desires for future you through crayons on paper.

You can also use magazines, newspaper cuttings or printed images that support future you. Stick them on to your paper or board to make a multifaceted collage or 'mood board'. Get creative and have fun. The only rule here is that there are no rules. It's your future self which you are free to create on paper as you best see fit. When your picture is complete, photograph it and put it somewhere where you can revisit it often.

Adopting a mindset of curiosity and openness can be key in figuring out just what suits you best. Be willing to experiment, whether through mindful meditation techniques, written affirmations or letters, drawings or vision boards. Any and all of these techniques can support alignment to future you and help to develop a roadmap enabling you to tap into more of your future potential. As you crystallise and clarify your life direction through courage and self-belief you will be more likely to commit to consistent action. This can gently nudge you into new ways of thinking and being in the world.

Telling yourself a different story about who you can be in the future reframes your sense of identity and realigns your actions with who you want to become. In addition, remember just how important a role the mind plays when it comes to your physical health. A more positive, optimistic mindset can make all the difference. Just think about the research in the Journal of the American Heart Association connecting optimism to a 35 per cent reduction in heart disease, or the positive influence of the placebo effect.[2]

Visualising your goals is an active demonstration of your intentional commitment to achieving them. It's a foundation for a self-fulfilling prophecy: a flourishing future version of you.

Your Relationship with Self and Others

Self-care is a gift to you and everyone who matters in your life.

Start (and end) your day well

Do you have a morning ritual, an intentional habit to start your day well? Perhaps it's a cold shower, a few moments of stillness in the garden as you sip your morning coffee or some written reflections in a journal?

With many competing demands and conflicting choices, life can get busy for all of us, which is why a morning ritual can be so helpful. The beginning of the new day is a time you can control and make your own. It is an opportune time for a self-care ritual to sustain you throughout the remainder of your day.

Learning from the lives of very wise people can be illuminating, and I have always been struck by the simplicity and consistent brilliance of Benjamin Franklin. Best remembered as one of the Founding Fathers of the USA, Franklin was also a writer, scientist, inventor, diplomat, publisher and political philosopher with a long list of significant discoveries and achievements. Every year for 25 years Franklin published an almanac; even today, it is a timeless classic full of practical advice and wise words that espouses the many benefits of having a routine rooted in ritual and simplicity.

The main difference between routine and ritual is the underlying significance, if there is any. A routine is a simple pattern of behaviour; for example, brushing your teeth. A ritual, on the other hand, is a regular practice that has some deeper significance or meaning in terms of connecting with who you are as a person.

The early morning is when you often feel most focused and free from the inevitable distractions and busyness of the day ahead. Having a morning ritual can help you to live more intentionally, more deliberately and with more purpose. It can provide a solid foundation to start your day and step forward grounded in presence.

While everyone is different, here's what I recommend to support you to start your day well.

Exercise

Get a few minutes of exercise shortly after you wake up. This may be aerobic (a brisk walk, run or cycle), some strength training, or simply stretching. The key idea is that moving gets your brain and body working better while burning off some cortisol, a stress hormone which is generally at its highest level first thing in the morning.

Embrace stillness

Next, take a few minutes of stillness and complete silence as a natural foil to the early morning workout. Starting the day with some stillness and silence can be a wonderful gift to your inner self, bringing peace of mind, mental clarity and emotional equanimity. The ritual of quiet reflection provides the focus and clarity needed to plan and subsequently execute your daily priorities.

Ensure your mobile devices are switched off as you find a quiet spot where you will be uninterrupted. While being outdoors in nature is ideal, even a view of nature can be very calming. Otherwise, simply sitting quietly in a chair can do the trick. This is an opportune time to reflect on your goals (for the day ahead, your year and life), your values and how you can serve others.

Be GLAD

Each day I do a short, written reflection using the mnemonic GLAD. It's my own personal morning ritual that prompts me to start my day well, grounded in gratitude and presence. The key is to take a few moments to reflect on each of the following questions. The answers can be brief – just a few intentional words that make a difference.

G: Good

What good will you do today?

Who can you encourage and support? What projects can you contribute to using your strengths and talents?

L: Looking forward to...

What are you looking forward to today?

Perhaps that lunch meeting or coffee conversation with a friend? Looking forward with a sense of anticipation is a wonderful way to bring more micromoments of positivity into your day to buffer any challenges later on.

A: Appreciation

Who can you appreciate today?

Think of someone who you can intentionally appreciate

through an active demonstration of gratitude or kindness. It might be something very small, perhaps the person who makes you that coffee. Active appreciation is in short supply nowadays. Buck that trend through your own actions. The smallest of positive actions can exceed the greatest of intentions.

D: Dedicated focus

What are you dedicating your time and energy to today? Are they your most important projects or goals, whether that's at work, at home or during your leisure time? And what distractions might derail these intentions if you are not careful?

What you focus your attention on tends to expand in your life. The key idea is that life, to a large degree, becomes how you choose to see it – whether you view it through the lens of gratitude and appreciation or the lens of absence and scarcity.

Get reading

For the final step in your morning ritual, I suggest reading. Read to learn, read to be inspired, read to enrich your mind. There are so many great books out there, more than anyone could hope to read in a lifetime. Personally I like to reread old favourites, books that ground me and support me in being my best self each day. Sometimes I will take a quote or line from a book that resonates with me at that moment, and to boost retention I write it in my journal. It is such a cathartic process to envision yourself becoming the tangible representation of those wonderful words. Words have tremendous capacity to inspire positive thoughts and emotions. When you commit those words to paper, they can embed inner confidence and positive change, deepening awareness and tuning you in to who you truly are.

What Went Well

Of course, just like a baton passed on in a relay race, ending your day well sets you up to start your day well tomorrow. As part of a nightly wind-down routine, consider this What Went Well ritual, or WWW. Developed by Dr Martin Seligman, often called the 'father of positive psychology', it acts as a reminder to focus on finding the good, on the sparks of light that can be found even among the dullest of days.

Consider: who or what inspired you today? What brought you happiness, comfort and deep peace today? What made you smile today? Did you make someone else smile? What brought you joy today? What projects did you make progress on? Did something go better than expected today? What positive conversations did you have? By focusing on these positive aspects of your life, you undertake a sort of filtering process, where you filter out the more irrelevant or negative events of the day.

End your day well by selecting those moments to savour that brought you joy and happiness. And on those tough days that we all experience, ask yourself: what did you learn? What can you still be grateful for? How can you grow? Was there a silver lining, enabling you to become a little wiser and stronger? As a ritual, WWW encourages you to better appreciate and savour positive events in the future. It is a great way to dissolve stress, broaden your perspective, and deepen gratitude, connection and meaning.

Fascinating research has found significant variations in the cellular mitochondria of caregivers. Those caregivers who start their day experiencing more positive emotions – or end their day with positive emotions – experience less stress, as evidenced by lower cortisol levels. In addition, they have higher levels of telomerase (an anti-aging enzyme) and better-functioning mitochondria.[1]

This demonstrates how experiencing positivity in the mind can show up in the body, providing further evidence of the mind–body connection. Positivity may manifest in various ways, such as a strong sense of purpose or meaning in one's caring role, gratitude or excitement, as well as positive emotions like joy or enthusiasm.

Starting your day well can be a wonderful way to proactively recalibrate your nervous system away from cortisol-soaked arousal and fight-or-flight, fear-based reactions. Instead, you can move toward present-moment awareness. Grounded in presence, and rooted in abundance and appreciation, you can step into your day more energised and alive to the rich potential it may bring.

As Gandhi once wrote so eloquently, your thoughts influence your words, which inspire your everyday choices and ultimately impact the direction of your life and your destiny. This is why your morning ritual is so important for your wellbeing. Committing to ritualising a great start to your day can lead to many positive consequences. You can build self-confidence, establish structure and gain a sense of control over your day, with a more upbeat attitude. This, in turn, lowers stress while boosting motivation, productivity and happiness. It allows you to reap the benefits of mood-boosting endorphins such as serotonin and noradrenaline while supporting positive mental health.[2]

Your morning and evening rituals can connect your long-term goals and aspirations with the actions you take starting today. What works best for you is simply what works best for you. There are so many potential rituals to choose from – whether it's cold showers, savouring great coffee, or even making your bed. I'm not suggesting you 'need' any particular one, and there is certainly no 'one size fits all' when it comes to daily rituals. My goal is simply to highlight the benefits of experimenting to figure out what suits you best.

Learning to prioritise the start and end of your day can make a huge difference: you'll feel calmer, more in control, and able to get much more done. Try creating your own morning and evening rituals to reframe your day for more presence, perspective and patience.

Make your bed

Modern living, with its throwaway culture, can lead to the accumulation of so much stuff and the result is so much clutter. Keeping on top of everything can feel like a full-time job at times, particularly for time-pressed parents and workers. Research from Princeton University has found that physical clutter can compete for your attention span just as multitasking does. This can increase feelings of frustration and toxic stress with a negative impact on mood. It can reduce performance and productivity, deplete willpower and dampen creativity.[1]

One of the problems with clutter is the visible reminder it provides that you are disorganised. It's an ongoing reminder of what you are not doing, which is a recognised downward drag on your wellbeing. By contrast, simplicity can unleash the potential of your subconscious mind to be heard more clearly, as you create space for new possibilities to emerge in your life.

Where, then, to begin? Easy – with making your bed. Yes, really! While it sounds like such a small step, the ritual of making your own bed can inspire self-confidence and inner calm and enhance your wellbeing.

Starting your day by making your bed can boost positivity and provide a sense of achievement. You embrace your day knowing that you have already accomplished one task, a 'micro-win'. This can trigger an upward spiral, energising, encouraging and empowering you to complete another task, and another. Many people believe that making their bed is an important aspect of starting the day well, leading to a day-long boost in productivity and a sense of achievement at the end of their day.

The visual impact of a neatly made bed dissipates feelings of stress, as the more ordered nature of your outer environment enhances inner calm. It grounds you in reality, making you feel more organised and better able to embrace the challenges of the day. As your organisational skills strengthen, you improve your ability to focus – a neatly made bed is a great start in the quest to declutter your space. By doing this, you can strengthen decision-making, support resilience and develop mental discipline through the action of making your bed – especially when you don't feel like it (on a dark winter morning, for example).

This little ritual can create a sense of calm and composure in the centre of your bedroom – the living space where you begin and end each day. This can conserve mental energy, enhance creativity and improve mental clarity. Furthermore, having a tidy living space is associated with being more conscientious and goal driven. All of this supports feelings of realistic optimism and overall life satisfaction.

By itself, the ritual of making your bed may seem mundane or menial, hardly worthy of any fuss or attention. However, making your bed signals an intention to your subconscious mind that you are serious about starting to declutter your space. Making your bed provides a tangible reminder that you can control how you start your day, instilling a feel-good sense of accomplishment before you've even had that first cup of coffee. This small act can ramp up your sense of motivation, which can cascade outwards into other aspects of your life. This may include being more generous, with some research finding that volunteers who filled out surveys in a messy room were less likely to want to donate to charity, compared to when the same surveys were completed in a tidy room.[2]

The bedroom is an important space, given that you spend about one-third of your life there. Tidying this space by making your bed in the morning is a positive intervention to your lived environment that can also enrich the positivity of your inner environment – by which I mean the space between your ears. Feelings of inner calm can ensue as a result. Furthermore, you are creating a restful, restorative space to return to each night, which may significantly increase your likelihood of a good night's sleep. This enables you to awaken more refreshed and recharged, with more zest and readiness for the day ahead.

Making your bed is a self-care ritual that builds awareness – awareness of your potential to choose order over disorder, simplicity over complexity and self-care over self-neglect. Awareness provides clarity to make more health-enhancing choices for your overall wellbeing. In terms of making your bed, your expanded sense of awareness can lead to a domino effect whereby you decide to clear up the rest of your bedroom, office, living space or car interior, etc. As we know, a decluttered space can be transformed into a space of tranquillity, creativity and serenity. You lower your feelings of stress, experiencing a sense of lightness and more presence. Making your bed may also be just the magic ingredient to spice up your sex life too! Sleep industry website Sleepopolis found that out of the 2,000 Americans surveyed, those who made their beds had sex once more per week on average than those who did not.[3]

Remember the sense of calm contentment when you see the crisply made bed in your hotel bedroom – how it boosts your mood. You can create a similar sanctuary in your own bedroom, one morning at a time.

I'll leave the last word on the benefits of making your bed to Naval Admiral William McRaven. In a famous commencement speech delivered at the University of Texas at Austin in 2014, he spoke about the benefits of making your bed first thing in the morning; how that small, simple ritual provides a sense of psychological security. Safe in the knowledge that you have already successfully completed one task, it creates a ripple effect of many more tasks being accomplished that day.

In his words: 'By the end of the day, that one task completed will have turned into many tasks completed.' An upward trajectory of incremental positive action, whereby one small ritual becomes the catalyst for further change.

Be your own best friend

Does your inner critic tend to run riot, telling you all the reasons why you aren't talented enough, young enough or successful enough? Do you have a perfectionistic mindset, where good enough is never quite good enough? Are you too tough on yourself? If so, you are not alone.

When I reflect on people who have grown up in the school of hard knocks and overcome significant life adversity, Liam is prominent in my mind. Orphaned at a young age, he was raised by an older sister who had her own serious mental health issues. For years, Liam struggled to accept what had happened to him. He blamed himself for his circumstances, taking refuge initially in work and, later on, in alcohol and prescription drugs. It was only after a broken marriage, bankruptcy and a battle with addiction that he began the long, slow journey to recovery.

As Liam himself said when reflecting on that period, 'My life was a mess. Things only started to get better once I faced up to the fact that while I couldn't change the past, I could stop it from poisoning the present moment, which it had done for years. I hated myself so much. I had blamed the world for all my woes. The day I started treatment was one of the best days of my life. It gave me a chance to start again, to see the world through fresh eyes. Through therapy, I learned to stop the self-sabotage and self-loathing. It gave me a chance to take responsibility for my own actions but, more importantly, to heal on the inside. Which meant I had to learn to like myself again; to treat myself with compassion and to understand that this didn't make me a weak person; to open up to my emotions; to realise how important it was to take good care of myself. I'm really grateful that I got that second chance.'

As a family doctor, you become a close confidante of your patients and the many experiences that life may bring to their door. With people busier and more stressed than ever in a world that's always 'on', holistic self-care is often neglected. If you are like most people, chances are that you could benefit from cultivating self-compassion and overall self-care.

Furthermore, for many people nowadays, social media opens the doorway to a world of relentless negative comparison, reinforcing beliefs you may have about why you don't quite measure up. Factor in the hardwired tendency to beat yourself up with self-criticism and you will begin to appreciate how important self-compassion and being kind to yourself really is.

Let's take a step back for a moment and remind ourselves just what compassion is, including the 'three As' of awareness, action and 'altogetherness'.

First, awareness that someone is struggling or suffering is the starting point for compassion. In other words, opening your eyes, heart and mind to being present and seeing the person and their situation as it really is. Easier said than done, of course, in a world of busyness and mindless distraction.

Secondly, as well as 'seeing' or 'feeling' someone's suffering, you are also moved to action. This 'action' is the main difference between compassion and empathy, which is simply feeling or experiencing someone's suffering. Through action, your heart responds to the other person's distress through a desire to help, assist or simply offer kindness and understanding as opposed to harsh judgement when someone slips up.

Thirdly, there is an 'altogetherness' about compassion. By this I mean a recognition and appreciation that everyone experiences tough times. No one is immune from loss, bereavement, illness or family issues, not to mention the many modern-day sources of toxic stress. Adversity is part and parcel of the shared experience of being human, encapsulated so eloquently by the old Sanskrit saying '*Vasudhaiva Kutumbakam*', meaning 'We are all part of the one human family.'

You are not a machine. The very definition of being human means that you are fragile, imperfect and vulnerable. Self-compassion is shining the light inwards and directing the 'three As' of compassion towards yourself. It's understanding that you are not a human *doing*, but a living, breathing human *being*. It's recognising how far you've already travelled in life, both in terms of your achievements and adversities overcome; it's better accepting and making peace with yourself, it's appreciating what and who you have in your life.

When you make a mistake or miss the mark, it can be so easy to start berating yourself with negative self-talk. With self-compassion, you give yourself the benefit of the doubt and treat yourself with more dignity and respect. You ask yourself, what might you say to your best friend if they approached you with a similar worry or concern?

Most likely you would give your friend patience, empathy, care, kindness and support. Now ask yourself how your best friend might support and help you in this very same situation. Almost certainly with the same encouragement, kindness, non-judgement and support. With self-compassion, you simply become your own best friend when you make a mistake, fail or stumble in life.

While positive self-talk is consistently celebrated as a means of reframing your mindset, the evidence for this remains weak at best. In fact, positive self-talk may actually do some harm by enabling you to deny reality, engage in a deception that everything is 'perfect' and suppress associated negative emotions.

Real self-talk provides encouragement rather than even more self-criticism. Encouragement is a wonderful word that comes from the French *en courage*, meaning 'with courage'. As a doctor, I've met many people over the years worn out by toxic workplaces, dysfunctional relationships or sometimes simply by life itself. I've never yet met someone who has come into my office and said they were being over-appreciated or over-recognised at work or in life.

Many people default to their inner critic mode when stressed or upset, as the emotional amygdala overwhelms your brain's capacity for a more rational response. Just like bricks in a wall, each additional brick of negative toxic self-criticism builds a wall of disconnection from your true self.

Trying to suppress these negative emotions or struggling to accept them tends to make matters much worse. In addition to feelings of sadness, you may feel guilty for feeling sad. As well as anxiety, you may feel angry for feeling anxious. Compounding stress, now you feel stressed for even feeling stressed. Self-compassion enables you to turn down or change the channel on this inner critic of self-recriminating judgement as you become more curious with your emotions rather than critical. As such, you are able to broaden and deepen your emotional reservoir.

In this way, self-compassion can be seen as a key element of any strategy of successful and sustainable self-care. In my opinion, the starting point for self-care is this 'inside-out' journey of seeing life through this lens of self-compassion. Practising self-compassion provides significant longer-term benefits for your current and future self. This includes being more aware of and attuned to your thoughts and emotions. You develop greater emotional agility, becoming more responsive and less reactive in your choices and decisions. You become more open, more trusting and kinder to others. It can even improve your sleep![1]

Self-compassion and kindness to yourself build a bridge to more sustainable self-care through your new commitment to value health, relationships and overall wellbeing. Higher levels of self-compassion are linked to increased feelings of curiosity, connectedness, happiness and optimism. In addition, it is associated with reduced ruminative thoughts and less anxiety, depression and fear of failure. As you become more confident and resilient, you support personal and professional growth while boosting overall life satisfaction. Self-compassion can move you away from the destructive self-sabotaging flaw-based focus of your inner critic to lightening up and living more at ease in your own skin.[2]

In a world where you can be anything, be kind to others, certainly, but please remember to be kind to yourself too. Accept and love yourself for who you are, focusing on your strengths, while empowering yourself to be authentically YOU. As a wise person once wrote, in the end, people will judge you anyway. So don't live your life trying to be liked by others. Live your life learning to love yourself!

Learn to let go

To feel wronged or mistreated – whether by family, friends or foes – is an almost universal experience. Life is rarely ever fair or plain sailing for anyone. At some stage, all of us will have minor slights or major grievances to contend with – and we will have to decide whether or not we can find forgiveness in order to let them go.

As a doctor I have met many people who struggle with this idea of 'letting go'. To experience anger is a completely normal part of the human emotional experience, but ongoing toxic anger about perceived injustice can be highly detrimental to your emotional, mental and physical wellbeing. Unresolved anger can trigger emotional pain which can consume everyday life. Research published in the *Journal of the American College of Cardiology* has highlighted that toxic anger and hostility are linked to both higher risk of heart disease and poorer outcomes for those people with existing heart disease. It can keep you stuck in a chronic fight-or-flight state of toxic stress, which negatively impacts your blood pressure, while increasing the risk of chronic health conditions such as diabetes, depression and heart disease. It can weaken your immune system, impacting your ability to fight off infection.[1]

Furthermore, chronically elevated levels of the stress hormone cortisol can have a corrosive effect on your hippocampus, the brain area responsible for turning experiences into lasting memories. This can keep you stuck in the past, unable to really enjoy the present moment. Thoughts of revenge and retribution can foster feelings of resentment, anger and even hatred – negative emotions that can prove tremendously toxic for your health and wellbeing. You may experience emotional disequilibrium and disconnection from your values and authentic self, creating a sense of spiritual poverty. In terms of your relationships, holding onto grudges can lead to a hangover effect whereby you bring anger and resentments forward into new relationships, negatively impacting their quality and durability, which can result in social isolation.

Forgiveness is defined as being able to release feelings of resentment or revenge towards a person who has harmed you, irrespective of whether they deserve it or not. It includes letting go or moving on, while also doing something positive towards the person that hurt you. This may involve an expression of empathy, communicating compassion or simply demonstrating an understanding of their situation or position. It is not about either denying or trivialising the seriousness of an incident or about letting someone 'off the hook'.

Forgiveness can work in three different ways. Firstly, forgiving someone else who has hurt you in some way; secondly, forgiving yourself for ways in which you have acted or behaved badly; and thirdly, forgiving a certain circumstance or situation not in your direct control (such as an accident, illness or loss). While this is not necessarily easy, through a process of acknowledging your pain and suffering and allowing the process of letting go, either by yourself or with professional help, you can take those first steps towards the gift of inner peace. You can choose to let go of past experiences or injustices, whether perceived or real. To look forward instead with confidence to a better, brighter future, free of resentment or feelings of recrimination.

Forgiveness is an action, an emotional choice, a character strength. It is a powerful construct in positive health and a virtue that values emotional freedom over emotional pain. It is neither excusing nor erasing bad memories. By intentionally choosing to let go, you exercise your right to remove any ongoing negative impact that person or situation has on your wellbeing. As a gift to your peace of mind, forgiveness prevents you from remaining chained to the suffering of the past.

Mark Twain once described forgiveness as 'the fragrance that the violet sheds on the heel that has crushed it'. Learning to forgive those who have hurt you can significantly improve your health and overall wellbeing. It is a key ingredient of inner peace, contentment and fulfilment and is an essential prerequisite to healing and spiritual growth.

While some people are naturally more forgiving than others, it's a skill that can be learned and improved upon. In a recent randomised controlled trial known as the International REACH Forgiveness Intervention, 4,598 participants from five countries were randomly assigned into two distinct groups.

The first group received a 'forgiveness workbook' which contained a number of expressive writing exercises. Each participant was tasked with describing a situation or specific incident that they hadn't forgiven through two separate lenses. Firstly, writing the story through the lens of your own experience. Secondly, through a more objective lens of an unbiased observer without any emotional context or feelings. As everyone sees things through their own worldview, writing through this window can boost understanding and relatedness, thereby potentially impacting forgiveness. Following these written exercises, the participants were asked to describe at least three differences they noticed between the two separate descriptions.

Compared to a control group who didn't participate, those who partook in the written exercises reported reduced symptoms of anxiety and depression while experiencing more feelings of forgiveness and more positive mental health and wellbeing.[2]

A recent study published in the *Journal of Health Psychology* suggests that forgiveness can act as a powerful protective buffer against the impacts of toxic stress on mental health, with the potential to alleviate stress, anxiety, hostility and low mood. It helps to rebalance the nervous system, creating calm and recalibrating the mind–body connection. The study assessed both the mental and physical health of 148 young adults. Not surprisingly, those with higher stress levels were found to have more health issues. However, the research also highlighted how in cases where participants expressed forgiveness (of others and of themselves) the association between stress and mental health issues was virtually eliminated.

Forgiveness can lighten the load of ruminating thoughts and reduce their negative impact. Forgiving someone can change how you see yourself and enhance your self-esteem. Physically, forgiveness can reduce pain perception and lower blood pressure and heart attack risk. It can improve sleep, immune health and mental wellbeing, and foster more robust relationships and overall life satisfaction, enabling you to live better and longer.[3]

As both a feeling and an action, forgiveness is a PRACTICE. If you want to bring more forgiveness into your life, here are some pointers which may be helpful:

P: Process

Forgiveness is an ongoing, active process – various hurts may need to be forgiven repeatedly as reminders surface and the associated emotions are recycled. It is always in your power to choose to respond with kindness, empathy and respect in the face of hurts or injustices perceived or real.

R: Remind

Remind yourself of the considerable benefits of expressing forgiveness for your own wellbeing – emotionally, mentally, relationally and physically. Remember to encourage yourself in your efforts.

A: Awareness

Forgiveness starts with awareness: awareness of what happened, how you felt at the time, how you reacted and how you feel now. Picture the issue and the person concerned clearly and objectively. Release any expectations of change. This heightened awareness can provide you with new clarity and insights to foster a spirit of forgiveness.

C: Choice

Forgiveness is your choice. You are choosing to let go and let be; you are choosing peace over anger, self-care over self-sabotage and healing over hurt.

T: Time Out

Consider time out to talk to someone you trust, gain a different perspective and strengthen your sense of self. You may want to try talk therapy with a trained therapist or support group, journalling and expressive writing, taking time to pray or meditating.

YOUR RELATIONSHIP WITH SELF AND OTHERS

I: If

If you are the person looking for forgiveness, remember to:

Acknowledge how your behaviour may have impacted others.

Avoid self-sabotaging destructive thoughts.

Ask for forgiveness genuinely and without making excuses.

Accept that whether you are forgiven or not is out of your hands.

C: Compassion

Compassion for others brings tolerance, gentleness and kindness to how you see people and situations. Remember that you may have been unfair to someone in the past who subsequently forgave you. Compassion for yourself is also important in order to release feelings of inadequacy or lack of self-worth if, or when, you are not treated well.

Putting yourself in someone else's shoes is a reminder that their actions may not have been personal to you and being empathetic can also reduce your own suffering. Instead of being judgemental, become curious about the circumstances that led the person to behave the way they did; perhaps you might even have acted similarly.

E: Emotional Agility

Don't repress or suppress your negative feelings. As you embrace the full spectrum of your emotions you become more emotionally agile, the hallmark of emotional freedom.

Ultimately you have a choice to make. Instead of staying trapped in a repetitive loop of negativity, you can choose to unburden yourself from the past actions of others. Engaging with forgiveness is not easy and some people are naturally more forgiving than others. The good news is that cultivating forgiveness as an ongoing self-care practice is a skill that almost everyone can learn and improve. The paradox of forgiveness is that as you let go of resentment and retribution towards someone else, you can experience significant wellbeing benefits yourself with healing, optimism and growth.

Instead of living in the prison of a grudge, you can build a bridge to a brighter, more flourishing future in an environment of emotional freedom. Choose the path of forgiveness and journey to a calmer, more peaceful, more hopeful place.

Avoid idle gossip

Journey to the Toshogu Temple in Japan and you will witness one of its most famous icons, a wooden statue of the three wise monkeys. Attributed to Confucius, who allegedly wrote to 'see no evil, hear no evil, speak no evil', they project a poignant message about the power of words.

The first monkey covers his mouth, symbolising the importance of not speaking ill of others or partaking in gossip, as to do so diminishes your karma and standing as a person. Likewise, the second monkey covers his eyes, reminding you to focus on that which is good and uplifting, rather than fixating on the negative which by extension drags you down as well. The third monkey covers his ears, which represents refusing to hear or listen to idle talk and thereby protecting your precious mind.

Humans have a well-known inclination to gossip. It's a fairly ubiquitous tendency that few may admit to liking but that almost everyone enjoys. Whether it's via WhatsApp group texts or workplace conversations, pretty much everyone who talks also talks about others, for better and (more often) for worse. Broadly defined as talking about other people who are not present at the time, gossip involves sharing information without permission. The information in question may of course be fun and fact-based or a fairytale of fictitious nonsense. Unfortunately, we tend to instinctively trust gossip, no matter how preposterous it sounds.

Hearing the word 'gossip' generally conjures up thoughts of malicious rumours, salacious stories or celebrity canoodling. It's incredibly prevalent as well, with research involving 467 participants published in the journal *Social Psychological and Personality Science* finding that the average person spends about 52 minutes per day gossiping. While about 75 per cent of the gossip was neutral in nature (typically conversational), 15 per cent was negative with only 9 per cent 'positive'.[1]

Often gossip is simply slander by another name and is inherently bad, having harmful consequences for the victim. Slander is essentially lying, whether you knowingly spread falsehoods or participate in the spreading of unconfirmed information about someone without the necessary evidence or proof. Sometimes people just jump to incorrect conclusions about people or events, and happily pass on misinformation. Perhaps this kind of gossip is triggered by envy, negative comparison or jealousy, or perhaps by real malevolent intent. Even being a passive participant in gossip can be enormously damaging. There is no doubt that gossip can destroy the lives of good people.

I was curious to research and learn more about the psychology of gossip. Is gossip always malicious, or can it be a good thing? Is it just rooted in jealousy and begrudgery or does it represent something else, perhaps a sort of 'groupthink' or herd mentality? If gossip is so potentially destructive, then why do so many people engage with it?

From an evolutionary standpoint, to successfully survive and pass on your genes it was necessary to not just be interested in but to have detailed knowledge of the lives of others in your space (friend and foe alike). Quite literally your life and very survival might depend on it, ergo the origins of gossip as an important survival tool. Imagine what life was like thousands of years ago for your hunter-gatherer ancestors; how their survival necessitated sharing information about safety and security, figuring out food sources and finding out who was dependable. Knowing who to trust and building trust strengthened the group overall. This ability to remember faces, names and the nuances of gossip enabled social groups to bond together and conferred a biological advantage. This makes intuitive sense, as being able to predict the probable behaviour of others based on knowledge of their personal habits was and remains advantageous today, both for survival and for life success.

Gossip impacts the brain too, with research using fMRI scans finding that gossip in general increased brain activity in the medial prefrontal cortex, an area involved in managing complex social emotions, with one of the brain's reward centres (the caudate nucleus) activated particularly in response to negative gossip about celebrities.[2]

Research published in the *Journal of Personality and Social Psychology* has highlighted the difference between passive and active participation in gossip. Passive participation, i.e., hearing about some antisocial behaviour or something negative about someone, triggers a mini stress response in your body as evidenced by an increased heart rate. By contrast, actively participating in the gossip – that is, telling someone else – lowered heart rate and helped calm the body (reversing the impact of hearing the initial negative gossip).[3]

Interestingly, those who spend considerable time negatively gossiping about others may themselves suffer from low self-esteem. Negative gossip may provide the gossiper with temporary distraction from feelings of stress, insecurity or anxiety.

Schadenfreude is a German expression for the pleasurable feelings of self-satisfaction that come from learning about the failings of another – when their pain becomes your gain! Perhaps it derives from social comparison, the idea of climbing the social status ladder when rivals experience bad fortune.

Studies using brain scans have found that schadenfreude correlates closely with the negative emotion envy. Experiencing strong feelings of envy towards an individual activated physical pain channels in part of the brain known as the dorsal anterior cingulate cortex. When that same individual suffers misfortune, the envious person experiences schadenfreude with activation in the reward centres of the brain such as the ventral striatum. The strength of the schadenfreude experienced was relative to the extent of the envy.

Relatability also matters when it comes to gossip. Research looked at the impact of students hearing news about a large inheritance or academic award. If it related to their peers, friends or partners, interest in this information was high with a significant chance of gossip spreading related to the news. By contrast, similar news about their professors was deemed to be of low interest with little chance of the news being spread.[4]

The exploitative potential of negative gossip to enhance social standing and social competition means gossip is often targeted at high-profile individuals and perceived rivals. Positive information doesn't tend to spread in the same way because it just doesn't serve the gossiper's own self-interest.

Here are some strategies to consider, what I term the 'Four As' to enable you to more effectively deal with negative gossip and avoid becoming an unwitting participant.

Awareness

Be aware: recognise when conversations are veering into destructive gossip, and also be aware of the impact the gossip has on you. While this may be subtle, there's no doubt that exposure to needless negativity can increase your feelings of toxic stress and reduce your subjective wellbeing. Just like a dry sponge immersed in water, your brain will soak up all its exposures. Make sure they're not unduly negative or you may experience collateral damage in terms of your emotional wellbeing. Stick to fact-based, constructive conversations.

Avoid

Avoid negative gossip if and where possible. Speak about more uplifting things. Adjust the frequency, or as I say, change the channel or the altitude of your language. Switch the topic of conversation to something neutral or a positive attribute about the person concerned and see how the tone can change.

Ask

Ask some reflective questions. Just what is the intention behind the negative gossiping about someone else? Is there a valid or compelling reason to share it? Is it being shared in order to damage someone else? How would you feel if someone else were to say something similar about you without a shred of evidence? What is the impact and potential harm of spreading unverified information?

Action

Politely decline to participate in gossip. Take affirmative action and address the gossiper directly, explaining that you don't feel comfortable listening to this and change the topic of conversation. Alternatively, ask if and how the gossiper proposes to help and support that person, through practical supports and steps. Show respect in your own speech and encourage others to do the same. Say unto others as you would like said unto – or about – you!

Of course, gossip can include neutral, negative, and positive information. At its best, gossip can be a social skill that frames you as a purveyor of valuable information and an encouraging team player. At its worst, it can be self-serving and salacious, damaging careers, destroying reputations and undermining relationships. The key, as with many things in life, is having the wisdom to appreciate and value the difference.

The art of great conversation is understanding the difference between words that are meaningful and uplifting and words that should never be spoken. Perhaps we should live by a saying that resonates loudly from my own childhood: 'If you've nothing nice to say, say nothing.' I'll leave the last word with Socrates, who, as we have learned, suggested that before you speak, you should filter your words through three separate questions. Is what you are about to say true, is it necessary and is it kind?

Have that friend you can call on, morning, noon or night

Jenny had always been something of an introvert. To the outside world, she appeared as a very independent person who lived alone and worked diligently in a local government office. Behind the scenes, however, that job was Jenny's only real connection to the outside world. Over time, Jenny's loneliness had created an emotional undertone of negativity that impacted her confidence, her decision-making and her sense of self.

One weekend while at the supermarket, Jenny developed a sudden feeling of tightness in her chest. Her head started to spin and she felt the world closing in around her. She was taken by ambulance to hospital, where a battery of tests found nothing physically wrong with her heart. Ultimately, a panic attack was the diagnosis, and she was prescribed a short course of Xanax to relax her. When I saw her in my office for a follow-up appointment the following week, Jenny opened up for the first time about how she really felt.

With time Jenny has come to understand how her loneliness was the root cause of her physical symptoms. She began to take some important baby steps toward reprioritising friendships and making an effort to reintegrate back into her community. She told me recently about how things changed for the better as she became intentionally more interested in others.

'I was never going to be the life and soul of the party,' Jenny said. 'I'm an introvert and like my own company. But I do understand and value the importance of human connection as well – particularly with people with shared interests, values and attitudes. My therapist also suggested that I reconnect with the things I feel passionate about. My whole life I've been interested in issues to do with social justice – it's probably the reason I ended up working in the civil service. So I started to volunteer with a local group that provided some shelter and hot food to the homeless. I got my spark back and it's made a big difference.'

Within a few months, Jenny found herself becoming part of a new network of people who shared a common interest. Becoming aware of how her loneliness was impacting her health, appreciating that she had the potential to make some changes and following through with positive actions has made all the difference.

Jenny's situation is far from unusual. Loneliness has become increasingly common, with at least one in every five people now reporting feeling disconnected, alone and isolated. An American Psychiatric Association Healthy Minds Monthly Poll conducted in early 2024 found that 30 per cent of adults experienced feelings of loneliness at least once a week over the past year, while 10 per cent felt lonely every day.[1]

The late John Cacioppo, a professor at the University of Chicago and a founder of the field of social neuroscience, spent a large percentage of his professional life studying loneliness. In his book *Loneliness: Human Nature and the Need for Social Connection*, he highlighted the increased prevalence of loneliness and its connection to changing norms in society, particularly the rise in individualism and increased numbers of people living alone. He also emphasised that the perceived stigma of loneliness being the result of a sort of character defect of being socially inadequate or shy could become a further barrier to people seeking help and support. Furthermore, he found that loneliness is contagious and can spread through social networks, particularly among friends.[2]

Research has found that feeling lonely triggers hyper-vigilance to social threat. Picking up on signs of social rejection or social threats more quickly leads to a vicious cycle of withdrawal which further intensifies feelings of isolation. This can result in a downward spiral, making it even more challenging for someone experiencing loneliness to reach out and build relationships even though that is what's most needed.

Of course, there is a world of difference between spending time alone and experiencing loneliness. Being alone can be a wonderful opportunity to disconnect from distractions, to reflect, relax and recharge. Some of the happiest and most fulfilled people on the planet spend considerable time alone and wouldn't consider themselves to be lonely for one second.

Loneliness on the other hand is an emotional response to the perception of being alone, excluded, apart from the crowd. Experiencing temporary loneliness from time to time is part and parcel of being human, particularly following a bereavement or a relationship break-down. However, extended periods of loneliness may be a symptom of a mental health issue such as depression or low self-esteem or, as in Jenny's case, indicative of an absence of supportive interpersonal relationships.[3]

Research using fMRI scans has found that social rejection lights up the same brain areas that are activated when we experience physical pain.[4] I see chronic loneliness as a pain that pervades every aspect of your wellbeing, negatively impacting your heart, mind, body and spirit. As a doctor, something that has really struck me is that persistent loneliness can have adverse health risks comparable to those from smoking cigarettes, obesity and high blood pressure. Social isolation and loneliness are associated with a 29 per cent increased risk of heart disease and a 32 per cent increased risk of stroke. Absence makes the heart grow fonder, as the saying goes, but it can also make the heart weaker! Loneliness increases levels of circulating stress hormones, which over many years put strain on your heart and blood vessels, increasing the risk of heart disease, blood clots and stroke. Being lonely can quite literally cause a broken heart![5]

Loneliness can trigger feelings of fatigue, increase your sensitivity to pain, trigger depression, make you less likely to adopt a healthy lifestyle and make you more likely to depend on alcohol. As you get older, loneliness increases risk of functional decline, falls, forgetfulness and increased biological ageing. The adverse health impacts of loneliness are significant, with a meta-analysis of 300,000 people finding that greater social connection is associated with a 50 per cent reduced risk of early death.[6]

The antidote to loneliness is human connection, reaching out to others and experiencing a sense of togetherness. Friends provide emotional satisfaction and support, strengthen sense of self and satisfy a deep need to belong, whether through common interests or shared purpose.

The Harvard Study of Adult Development is the longest in-depth longitudinal study of human life ever done. Starting in 1938 during the American Great Depression, it continues to evolve and expand as it now includes the descendants of the original participants. What is truly brilliant about this research is that from the very start, it focused on understanding human health through the lens of being well rather than simply beating illness; thriving and flourishing, as opposed to simply surviving; what's strong as opposed to what's wrong. In other words, the essence of what's now widely recognised (but was not yet described back then) as positive health and positive psychology.

At the beginning, it compared 238 first-year Harvard college students (including a certain future president John F. Kennedy) with young men in the inner city of Boston who lacked the traditional trappings of a comfortable life. Women weren't included in the original study group as college entry at that time was all male. These groups and their offspring (now including women) have been painstakingly followed up since that time, providing a wealth of data pertaining to potential influences on physical and mental health.

What's fascinating is that the unfolding lives of the study participants have been studied in real time through the taking of hundreds of measurements and the asking of thousands of questions. While several factors including fitness, food and fulfilment from career impact on long-term health, none of these factors come close to the importance of positive relationships. The Harvard Study has found that those people most satisfied with their relationships at age 50 turned out to be the healthiest at age 80. George Valiant, Director of the Harvard Study of Adult Development for many years, described relationships as a 'master strength', having that capacity to love and be loved.

His question for you was this: 'Have you got someone you feel comfortable phoning at five o'clock in the morning to tell your troubles to?' His rationale was that answering 'yes' to that question meant you were far more likely to live longer than if the answer was 'no'.

Meitheal is an old Irish word that describes the coming together of a community to work in unity. This is perhaps traditionally best exemplified in the farming world at harvest time, where an individual might find it next to impossible to harvest their crop alone. However, when everyone works together all crops can be harvested.

Everyone succeeds with mutually beneficial outcomes, a real win-win. I really like the concept of the word *meitheal*, and the word contains both 'me' and 'heal' – a reminder that when we help each other we also help ourselves.

STAYING CONNECTED: NINE WAYS TO MAINTAIN A HEALTHY FRIENDSHIP

1. Just as a plant in a garden needs to be cultivated, so do your friendships need investment of time and energy.
2. Treat others as you would like to be treated. Be dependable, follow through on your commitments and keep your promises.
3. Be an encourager. Focus on the strengths of your friends rather than their faults. Speak well of them in their absence.
4. Create time and space for mutually enjoyable experiences – sharing a meal, watching a match together, going to the gym, volunteering.
5. Become a better listener. Be fully present when you're together by putting away your devices and limiting distractions. Be empathetic and non-judgemental. Listen to understand rather than respond. Embrace silence as a space for deeper, richer connections.

6. Check in regularly, whether through a quick text, a call or an in-person meetup.
7. Remember that small, thoughtful gestures can add up to make a big difference. Show your friends that they're important to you.
8. Offer practical and emotional support during challenging times – think stressful life events, relationship breakups or job changes.
9. Share moments and build memories by celebrating milestones and achievements together.

A wise man once said to be grateful for your friends, for they are the gardeners that make your soul blossom. Of course, it's easy to neglect your friends as relationships require investment of time and effort. While the best time to plant a tree was 30 years ago, the next best time is today. What are some seeds you can sow today to nurture existing friendships or develop new ones? If you want more friends in your life, be more friendly. If you want more support in your life, be more supportive. If you want more connection in your life, reach out and connect more with others. Taking action to nurture and strengthen your relationships is something that your future self will thank you for!

Embody the spirit of *amor fati*

Do you consider yourself to be Stoic?

The word might initially seem irrelevant, perhaps even meaningless, to you – or it may evoke ideas of hardship and struggling in silence. For me, the word 'stoic' (spelt with a small 's') evokes images of surviving tough times with self-deprecating suffering. This mindset, character-ised by oppression combined with passivity, was some-thing many generations of Irish people were conditioned to accept. It reminds me of the resignation depicted in stories like that of Peig Sayers, familiar to many Irish adults from their school days. Silence was central to this stoic mindset – not complaining about things, but equally not doing much to change them, either because of one's circumstances or the self-image shaped by them.

So, you might wonder: why would your future self thank you for living your life by this approach?

The key lies in the spelling. While the *Oxford English Dictionary* defines 'stoicism' as 'the endurance of pain or hardship without the display of feelings and without complaint', Stoicism (with a capital 'S') is an Ancient Greek school of philosophy – and it's a philosophy that I believe your future self will deeply appreciate.

The term Stoic originates from the Greek word 'stoa,' meaning 'porch'. It was on porches that people once gathered to hear the philosopher Zeno speak about vision and values. Vision refers to how you choose to interpret events – rather than the events themselves – which often becomes the root of much unhappiness. Values such as courage, self-control, justice and wisdom can lead to lasting well-being. Traits of a Stoic philosopher include honesty, integrity, cheerfulness in the face of obstacles, willpower, indifference to trivial matters, and finally calm, rational decision-making. Stoics value reason above all else.

Although the Stoic philosophers lived long ago, their wisdom endures. I first encountered the Stoics after the fire that destroyed my practice premises. During the great financial crash, this outlook was invaluable in supporting patients when fear and financial stress left many feeling broken. People were seeking new ways to cope, and in my search to help others, I found some of the oldest ideas ever written. These teachings have profoundly shaped my mindset, and I believe they can do the same for you. Everyone faces emotionally stressful times, with challenges never far from the horizon. Whether related to health, career, family, relationships or finances, life is rarely smooth sailing for long. This is where Stoicism comes in – not just as a way to navigate life's storms, but as a skill for personal growth. It offers a pathway to resilience, meaning and wisdom.

One person who benefited from these ideas was Peter, an optimistic, kind man with a love of sun holidays. He was an infrequent patient until he faced a health scare that changed everything: a dark mole on his chest was diagnosed as a melanoma. Alongside this frightening diagnosis, Peter was dealing with family troubles: his wife's long-standing conflicts with her parents, which had begun to affect his own family, and an 18-year-old son who had been binge drinking and who had recently ended up in the emergency department. Peter was overwhelmed and needed support. Among several self-care strategies, the idea of keeping a written journal resonated with him. He had always appreciated quotes and affirmations, and now he had the chance to take back control of his life through daily journalling.

Six months later, Peter was in a much better place. Thanks to early detection, his cancer required no further treatment beyond regular monitoring. He had encouraged his wife to seek help, which had improved their relationship with their son, who was now preparing for college. More importantly, Peter had been able to take stock of his life, using the insights gained from journalling to build a brighter future. In his own words, 'Writing down my experiences allowed me, for the first time, to step back and see things with fresh eyes. It's been a game changer, something simple yet powerful, helping me live more in the present while also planning for the future.'

This brings us to a core tenet of Stoic philosophy: *amor fati*, or the love of one's fate. It's the idea that you can embrace everything that happens – not with passive resignation, but with active acceptance. *Amor fati* involves not just accepting what is happening now, but embracing all that has happened and will happen. This mindset helps cultivate inner peace and contentment.

What separates humans from animals is our ability to choose how to respond in any given moment. This power of choice gives us incredible freedom. Rather than dwelling on doubt, despairing over weakness, or wallowing in self-pity, it's far better to focus on your strengths. Every obstacle can become an opportunity to face adversity with detachment and strength, enabling you to step forward with purpose into the future.

Journalling is a key strategy embraced by the Stoics. While you can't change the past, you can change how you interpret it. Almost every evening, Marcus Aurelius wrote in his journal about how to be more just, humble, empathetic and wise. His *Meditations* are a personal reflection on how to grow stronger and wiser, and they show what a worthy leader he was. Journalling can be a powerful tool for self-care, offering insights that also support your compassion for others.

There is something inherently powerful about writing things down. When you connect your brain through your hand to the journal, what you express in writing becomes impressed in your heart and mind. This act of handwriting stimulates multiple regions of the brain, helping you retain information and deepen your learning. The process gives you a cognitive edge – like 'thinking on paper'. Writing things down allows you to see life's challenges more clearly and objectively, and to reshape your future.

Keeping a journal can help you better understand yourself. The philosophers of old, even in an era without technology, understood that knowing oneself is key to living an enlightened life. To know who you are today, and more importantly, who you are becoming, strengthens self-awareness, self-acceptance and self-reflection.

Journalling also supports better decision-making, providing a safe space to consider the pros and cons of important choices. Over time, your journal becomes an accountability partner, recording your progress and encouraging self-improvement. As you get better at describing life to yourself, you also improve at describing yourself to life.

The emotional release from journalling helps prevent toxic emotions from spilling into your outer life. It can be cathartic, helping you build resilience and long-term well-being. Writing about fears diminishes their power, and writing about joy deepens your appreciation of life.

Above all, the Stoic approach encourages us to embrace change and take the right actions. By reframing your experiences through a growth mindset, you can become a little wiser and stronger. As Epictetus asked, 'How long are you going to wait before you demand the best for yourself?' Answering this question today is something your future self will undoubtedly thank you for.

Remember, one day you will die

Have you thought about your own mortality recently? Do you ever take a moment to acknowledge the inescapable truth that you will die one day? If you are like most people, then this thought is one of the furthest things from your mind – and understandably so. The architecture of your brain is fundamentally designed for danger detection and survival, not for dwelling on your own expiration date. Thoughts of the impermanence of life and your eventual demise and death may seem counterintuitive – and they make for a fairly morbid topic of conversation.

Fear of dying can trigger an intense fight-or-flight response, which is why this topic tends to be avoided like the proverbial plague. And yet, at the same time, death is all around us. Turn on the news and there are relentless reminders of tragic accidents, acts of terror and natural disasters. Closer to home, whether it's a personal health scare, illness or the death of a friend, neighbour or loved one, reminders of mortality are never far away.

In 2006, life presented me the opportunity to purchase, restore and convert an old Pugin-designed convent building (originally built in the 1840s) into a state-of-the-art primary care centre. When it opened in 2009 after extensive renovation and construction, it was a dream come true for me. Located quite literally 'up the road' from where I had grown up and renamed as the Waterford Health Park, it provides a range of primary healthcare services to this day, from family practice to pharmacy. Flooding the building with natural light created a warmer, more welcoming sense of place while staying sensitive to its original design. As an internationally recognised example of 'generative space' – an environment that is health-enhancing by design – it has attracted visitors from all over the world. In addition to an internal 'healing' garden, it has a coffee shop that focuses on food that is organic and plant-rich. The former chapel area is preserved in its original state and adorned with spectacular stained-glass windows. Look closely at their colourful patterns, however, and you may be surprised (as I was) to see several skull bones depicted in the lower aspects of the detailed designs. Curious to learn more about their meaning and symbolism, I discovered that the depiction of skull bones has been an integral part of art and architecture throughout history. They provide a graphic reminder of the fact that one day, we will all die – also known as a *'memento mori'*. This is a Latin phrase meaning 'remember you must die'.

It is an indisputable fact that death is the one thing guaranteed for each and every one of us, irrespective of whether you are currently young or old, healthy or unwell. It's inevitable and inescapable. Furthermore, remembering that one day you will die can become a powerful reminder to live more fully right now.

Hospice nurse and author Bronnie Ware has worked with hundreds of terminally ill patients during the last three months of their lives. In her book, *The Top Five Regrets of the Dying*, she beautifully captures the most common regrets at the end of someone's life.[1]

THE FIVE MOST COMMON END-OF-LIFE REGRETS

'I wish I'd had the courage to live a life where I was true to myself, and not just lived up to other people's expectations.'

'I wish I hadn't worked so hard.'

'I wish I'd had the courage to express my feelings.'

'I wish I'd stayed in better touch with my friends.'

'I wish I'd let myself be happier.'

Of course, we can experience regret at any stage in our lives, not just on our deathbeds. Mistakes are part and parcel of being human, after all. Perhaps the best thing to do about regret is to become really curious about it. It may signal an area of your life where there is potential for change or growth.

One of the most fascinating guests to appear on my podcast *In the Doctor's Chair* was Dr Akil, a family physician based in Alabama and the author of *Open Heart*. I first introduced you to Dr Akil in the 'Let your lifestyle be your medicine' chapter. He described his growth and new appreciation for life having experienced a near-fatal cardiac event at the age of 60. Aged 72 at the time of our interview, he described himself as being 'only twelve', such was the profound nature of his mindset shift. He has courageously chosen to take back control of his life and health journey, embracing life as a more active participant in his own wellbeing with a concrete plan to live more fully. His story is far from unusual; many people who have encountered near-death experiences describe profound change after the event. They tend to become more mindful, with greater immersion in their own lives as an authentic reflection of their true selves and their values. They tend to lose their fear of death, gaining a renewed sense of self and strengthened sense of spirituality. They also become more tolerant, open and caring, with a deeper sense of purpose and meaning.

But you don't need to experience a brush with death to awaken to the magical mystery of your life. You can start this today by cultivating awareness, which is the starting point for all meaningful change. New awareness and acceptance of the inevitability of death can create the mental space to reframe your mortality, inspiring you to live with more vitality. This can support your spiritual, psychological and emotional growth, enhancing your sense of self-esteem and overall wellbeing and sparking more appreciation for who and what you have in your life right now.

Courage is not the absence of fear – it's being willing to walk towards your fears in pursuit of something mean-ingful for you. You can face your fears around the inev-itability of death through finding the courage to live the life you want for yourself and not the life that others wanted for you. Remembering that you will one day die can inspire and empower you to live your best life authentically and more intentionally. It can encourage you to follow your dreams and foster stronger, more meaningful relationships. Moreover, it can gift you the wisdom to live more fully in the present moment, to have a crystal-clear vision of your life purpose and to value your time by treating each day as the precious gift it really is.

The Persian writer Saadi put it so well when he wrote, 'I bemoaned the fact I had no shoes until I saw the man who had no feet.' Can you think of someone you know who is less fortunate than you right now, someone who is perhaps experiencing serious illness, bereavement or personal difficulties? Focus on how fortunate you are that you do not have their particular challenges at this moment in time. Positive comparison in this way provides a reminder of just how precious life is, bringing more depth to your everyday experiences, enabling you to better appreciate life's giftedness.

In his letter 'On the Shortness of Life', the Stoic Seneca reminds us of just how valuable and limited your greatest resource – your time – really is. He writes, 'We are not given a short life, but we make it short, and we are not ill-supplied but wasteful of it.' Reflecting on the brevity of time provides a perfect antidote to many of life's so-called stressors.

Awareness of just how finite a resource time is can support you to make better choices in deciding how to spend it. So, value your time, and have no regrets. To counteract '*mañana* syndrome', the illusion of there being endless tomorrows, take action on those things that matter today.

A wise patient once remarked to me that a funeral cortège never has a trailer in tow containing the worldly possessions of the deceased. Death is the great equaliser, and there is simply no point in being the richest man in the cemetery given that both the prince and the pauper eventually turn to dust.

You don't need to wait for the wake-up call of a serious health scare or near-death experience to embrace life more fully. Simply bring a tangible reminder that you can touch and see into your everyday environment to connect with your own *memento mori*. Whether a pebble, rusty coin, or favourite saying, this simple reminder can inspire and propel you forward to live more fully, day in and day out.

You, like all of us, have an unknowable period of time left to live. So to use another Latin phrase, *carpe diem* – seize the day. Instead of just counting time, make your time count!

Build a bridge to future you

The poet Robert Frost once wrote, 'Two roads diverged in a wood, and I— / I took the one less travelled by, / And that has made all the difference.' At every stage of your life to date, you have made choices that have impacted your future self – for better and, at times, for worse. Sometimes you make choices that your future self may well regret; think relationships that run out of road and habits that have less-than-healthy consequences.

When I begin to imagine the exciting benefits that positive future change represents, my thoughts turn to the butterfly. We have had two beautiful sculptures of butterflies in the Waterford Health Park for many years to symbolise transformation, community and connection. They serve as a reminder of the potential within each one of us to choose the higher ground when it comes to our future health and wellbeing.

Of course, while we can admire the beauty of the butterfly, he certainly didn't begin his life like that. As Maya Angelou wisely wrote, 'We delight in the beauty of the butterfly, but rarely admit the changes it has gone through to achieve that beauty.' For a long time, the butterfly was a simple caterpillar, crawling around and consuming cabbage leaves. Thanks to imaginal cells deep within him, primitive impulses prompt him to leave the security of the ground to attach himself upside down to a leaf, twig or the branch of a tree, whereupon he starts to spin his chrysalis. Once ensconced safely inside, the process of transformation begins as he literally digests himself, until only a few cells, known as imaginal discs, remain. Once the eyes, body, legs, wings and antennae fully develop, the cocoon ruptures, enabling the butterfly to emerge, spread his wings and fly.

The Greek word for butterfly is *psyche*, meaning 'soul'. Metaphorically speaking, the butterfly represents that sense of soulful possibility that exists within all of us. An inner knowing that growth and positive change is possible. If you choose to remain as a caterpillar in life, you consume everything around you, including the emotions, environments and expectations of others. Too often these emotions are negative, environments health-depleting and expectations limited. In this way the caterpillar can become trapped, a victim of circumstance.

Before you start to spin your chrysalis, you need to be willing to let go of what you have or how you are seen by the outside world. This is the only way to become who you truly are. A prerequisite for this journey of transformation is courage: the courage to be true to yourself and your values; the courage to commit to those things that matter most; the courage to let go of what others may think or say about you; the courage to simply start. Perhaps most importantly, you must have the courage to keep one eye firmly on the future while continuing to live fully today.

While the caterpillar and butterfly are completely different versions of the same insect, your current and future self are different versions of you, too. You have the opportunity to become more aligned and attuned to that future you, while at the same time embracing the richness of present-moment awareness. You can become more alive, free from stagnation and the shackles of the past, free to spread your wings and face the future with boundless optimism – one day and one breath at a time.

More often than not, today's temptations take precedence over tomorrow's plans. This is a key reason why diets and other forms of denial tend to be sacrificed on the altar of instant gratification. Think about the gap between tipsy Saturday-night excitement and hangover-induced Sunday-morning existential angst and it's clear that the 'night before' version of you didn't consider how the 'morning after' version might feel. It can be hard to appreciate just how your everyday choices compound to create your future, for better and for worse. As Chinese philosopher Lao Tzu wisely mused thousands of years ago: 'Watch your thoughts; they become words. Watch your words; they become actions. Watch your actions; they become habits. Watch your habits; they become character. Watch your character; it becomes your destiny.'

If future you seems very different to who you are today – a distant stranger – then you are far more likely to favour short-term gain and instant gratification. If, however, you relate more closely to your future self, then you will be far more likely to make positive choices now that support this future version of you later.

Taking a bird's-eye view of time can change your perspective, helping you to see life events as a continuum – a constant flow without rigid boundaries between past or present or future.[1] As the Buddha wrote, 'Drop by drop is the water pot filled. Likewise, the wise man, gathering it little by little, fills himself with good.' Similarly, drop by drop, day by day you continue to evolve into your future self – for better and for worse.

No relationship, of course, is perfect. The vicissitudes of life ensure valleys and peaks for everyone. 'Staying in contention' is a term I frequently use to encourage patients with their health plans. Rooted in self-compassion, it gives you space to accept the reality of imperfection, to acknowledge and learn from setbacks while encouraging your efforts to get back on track. To never stop starting along this road less travelled. Stay committed to this relationship with yourself, with all its messy imperfections. Your future self will thank you for staying the course.

Recently, a friend shared a personal story that really resonated with me. His father was a primary school teacher in a rural part of Ireland, who had worked diligently all his life while raising his family. Back in the 1950s, Ireland was a poor country and travel was a luxury reserved for the privileged few. As he approached retirement, my friend's father spoke excitedly about his plans to travel abroad. With his family reared and mortgage cleared years earlier, he was looking forward to the day when, in his own words, he would be finally free to travel. And so, when his sixty-fifth birthday arrived, he decided to drive to Dublin to collect his retirement cheque – it meant that much to him.

Tragically, on the drive home later that evening, and through no fault of his own, he was involved in a fatal road traffic accident. Hit head on by a truck, he died instantly at the scene. My friend, at the time in his early twenties, recalls that day vividly. He was asked to identify the body and collect his father's few possessions. He remembers the cheque – not the amount, but the fact that it was bloodstained.

More than anything, this story is a poignant reminder that despite our best plans and intentions, the future for any of us is far from certain. No one knows how much time they have left, whether days or decades. Committing to being more present to those things that matter most to you can help ensure that you waste less of the precious time you have been given.

One of the real challenges with this idea is that living for a better future often means suspension of the present through various forms of delayed gratification. When you postpone present purchases or pleasures, you sacrifice the (guaranteed) present for the (unknowable) future. On the other hand, if you spend your life exclusively focusing on the future, you will miss out on the moments and experiences that create memories in your future. In the end it's a trade-off: live now, certainly, but keep one eye on the future as well.

As a teenager, one of my favourite films was *Back to the Future*. Michael J. Fox starred as the high school student Marty McFly, whose fortunes ebbed and flowed wildly as he travelled through time in a DeLorean time machine, alongside the eccentric scientist Doc Brown.

To my teenaged self, the concept that one could travel backwards or forwards in time was fascinating. One of the main themes was the idea of personal responsibility – that small choices and decisions made today can profoundly influence your future destiny.

While you can't physically travel through time, in the mind's eye you can. Thanks to part of the brain known as the default mode network or DMN, you can rapidly bounce from past to future and back to the present through 'thought travel'. Martin Seligman, a pioneer of positive psychology, describes this ability as a key ingredient of human thriving – that by being able 'to contemplate the future, we thrive by considering our prospects'. This supports you in staying on the path of self-improvement and self-realisation; choosing more wisely, leading to a healthier and happier, more vitalised future version of you.

Writing this book has been a real joy for me. It has reminded me to continue to view health and wellbeing through the lens of the future self and to never stop starting; to live in the here and now, while also embracing future me with more openness and optimism than ever. My hope is that it does the same for you too. To quote Doc Brown in *Back to the Future Part III*, 'Your future is whatever you make it, so make it a good one.'

Afterword:

Choose courage

Courage is one of six virtues that are common to all civilisations and cultures, going back for centuries. It sits alongside justice, humanity (or love), wisdom, temperance and transcendence. As such it is recognised as a key character strength, presenting variously as integrity, bravery or enthusiasm.

Just as positive health, emotional agility and flourishing include the reality of negative emotions and tough times, courage is not the absence of fear. Rather it represents a commitment through action to move towards those fears in pursuit of something that matters to you.

Charting and navigating a better course to future you starts with courage.

Courage is values over valuables.

Courage is action over words.

Courage is sometimes finding the words.

Courage is living your most real and authentic life.

Courage is holding space for vulnerability.

Courage is trusting (again).

Courage is opening your heart after the pain of rejection.

Courage is opening your mind to new ideas and fresh perspectives.

Courage is moving forward despite many defeats.

Courage is fear walking.

Courage is having the strength to carry on through the darkest days of despair.

Courage is being able to say goodbye to the past and the way things were while welcoming change and new beginnings.

Courage is letting go of the fixed beliefs that held you back.

Courage focuses less on mindless distraction and more on mindful doing.

Courage gets things done.

Courage gives freely without expectation.

Courage is living imperfectly.

Courage is loving fully.

Courage is facing the changes that ageing brings.

Courage is being able to ask for help.

Courage is finding a way back.

Courage says 'no' to good things to say 'yes' to better things.

Courage can allow you to be more fully present to life's realities.

Courage helps you to choose self-compassion over self-sabotage.

Courage is the inner knowing that right now, you are enough.

Courage is being vulnerable.

Courage is being able to change your mind.

Courage is being wrong and apologising.

Courage is admitting to not knowing.

Courage is celebrating life's little things.

Courage is staying a learner, a beginner, being willing to never stop starting.

Courage is sometimes a roar, sometimes a whisper.

Choose courage. Your future self will thank you for it.

Acknowledgements

Thank you to Gill Books for partnering with me again on my latest book. To Sarah Liddy for her confidence in me as a writer. To all the team, especially Aoibheann, for her professionalism and enthusiasm.

To Kerri Ward for her insightful editing and helpful suggestions.

To so many of my patients who have encouraged and supported me in my own journey to become a better advocate for positive health.

To friend and fellow author Abraham Verghese, for his kindness in writing such a favourable review for me.

Finally, to my wife Edel, whose unfaltering encouragement has been a real spark for my creativity. And to my three children: Malcolm, Tony and Lydia. My future self rests in you.

Endnotes

Introduction: Say hello to future you

1 Gilbert, D. (2014, March). *The psychology of your future self* [Video]. TED Conferences.

Leverage the science of habits

1 Lally, P., van Jaarsveld, C. H. M., Potts, H. W. W., & Wardle, J. (2010). How are habits formed: Modelling habit formation in the real world. *European Journal of Social Psychology*, 40(6), 998–1009. https://doi.org/10.1002/ejsp.674

2 Wood, W., Quinn, J. M., & Kashy, D. A. (2002). Habits in everyday life: Thought, emotion, and action. *Journal of Personality and Social Psychology*, 83(6), 1281–1297. https://doi.org/10.1037/0022-3514.83.6.1281

3 Martiros, N., Burgess, A. A., & Graybiel, A. M. (2018). Inversely active striatal projection neurons and interneurons selectively delimit useful behavioural sequences. *Current Biology*, 28(4), 560–573. https://doi.org/10.1016/j.cub.2018.01.008

Your Physical Health and Wellbeing

Become the CEO of your own health

1 National High Blood Pressure Education Program. (2004). *The Seventh Report of the Joint National Committee on Prevention, Detection, Evaluation, and Treatment of High Blood Pressure.* Bethesda, MD: National Heart, Lung, and Blood Institute (US).

2   SPRINT Research Group. (2015). A randomized trial of intensive versus standard blood-pressure control. *New England Journal of Medicine, 373*(22), 2103–2116. https://doi.org/10.1056/NEJMoa1511939

3   Brunner, F. J., Zeller, T., et al. (2019). Application of non-HDL cholesterol for population-based cardiovascular risk stratification: Results from the Multinational Cardiovascular Risk Consortium. *The Lancet, 394*(10215), 2173–2183. https://doi.org/10.1016/S0140-6736(19)32519-3

Eat fewer ultra-processed foods

1   Martini, D., Godos, J., Bonaccio, M., Vitaglione, P., & Grosso, G. (2021). Ultra-processed foods and nutritional dietary profile: A meta-analysis of nationally representative samples. *Nutrients, 13*(10), 3390. https://doi.org/10.3390/nu13103390

2   Lane, M. M., Gamage, E., Du, S., Ashtree, D. N., McGuinness, A. J., Gauci, S., et al. (2024). Ultra-processed food exposure and adverse health outcomes: Umbrella review of epidemiological meta-analyses. *BMJ, 384*, Article 3907. https://doi.org/10.1136/bmj-2023-074907

3   Juul, F., Vaidean, G., Lin, Y., Deierlein, A. L., & Parekh, N. (2021). Ultra-processed foods and incident cardiovascular disease in the Framingham Offspring Study. *Journal of the American College of Cardiology, 77*(12), 1520–1531. https://doi.org/10.1016/j.jacc.2020.12.051

4   Centers for Disease Control and Prevention. (2024, January). Get the facts: Added sugars. *CDC Nutrition.* https://www.cdc.gov/nutrition/data-statistics/added-sugars.html

5   Paterson, K. E., Myint, P. K., Jennings, A., Bain, L. K. M., Lentjes, M. A. H., Khaw, K. T., & Welch, A. A. (2018). Mediterranean diet reduces risk of incident stroke in a population with varying cardiovascular disease risk profiles. *Stroke, 49*(10), 2415–2420. https://doi.org/10.1161/STROKEAHA.118.021296

6   Martínez-González, M. A., Gea, A., & Ruiz-Canela, M. (2019). The Mediterranean diet and cardiovascular health. *Circulation Research, 124*(5), 779–798. https://doi.org/10.1161/ CIRCRESAHA.118.313348

Take cold showers and hot saunas

1   Esperland, D., de Weerd, L., & Mercer, J. B. (2022). Health effects of voluntary exposure to cold water: A continuing subject of debate. *International Journal of Circumpolar Health, 81*(1), Article 2111789. https://doi.org/10.1080/22423982.2022.2111789

2   Buijze, G. A., Sierevelt, I. N., van der Heijden, B. C. J. M., Dijkgraaf, M. G., & Frings-Dresen, M. H. W. (2018). Correction: The effect of cold showering on health and work: A randomized controlled trial. *PLOS ONE, 13*(8), e0201978. https://doi.org/10.1371/journal.pone.0201978

3   Salonen, J. T., Seppänen, K., Rauramaa, R., & Salonen, R. (1989). Risk factors for carotid atherosclerosis: The Kuopio Ischaemic Heart Disease Risk Factor Study. *Annals of Medicine, 21*(3), 227–229. https://doi.org/10.3109/07853898909149020

Enjoy great coffee

1   Chieng, D., et al. (2022). Regular coffee intake is safe and associated with improved mortality in prevalent cardiovascular disease and/or arrhythmia. *Heart, Lung and Circulation, 31*(S225). https://doi.org/10.1016/j.hlc.2022.07.372

2   van Dam, R. M., Hu, F. B., & Willett, W. C. (2020). Coffee, caffeine, and health. *New England Journal of Medicine, 383*(4), 369–378. https://doi.org/10.1056/NEJMra1816604

3   Ding, M., Bhupathiraju, S. N., Satija, A., van Dam, R. M., & Hu, F. B. (2014). Long-term coffee consumption and risk of cardiovascular disease: A systematic review and a dose-response meta-analysis of prospective cohort studies. *Circulation, 129*(6), 643–659. https://doi.org/10.1161/ CIRCULATIONAHA.113.005925

4   Crippa, A., Discacciati, A., Larsson, S. C., Wolk, A., & Orsini, N. (2014). Coffee consumption and mortality from all causes, cardiovascular disease, and cancer: A dose-response meta-analysis. *American Journal of Epidemiology, 180*(8), 763–775. https://doi.org/10.1093/aje/kwu194

5   Ding, M., Bhupathiraju, S. N., Chen, M., van Dam, R. M., & Hu, F. B. (2014). Caffeinated and decaffeinated coffee consumption and risk of type 2 diabetes: A systematic review and a dose-response meta-analysis. *Diabetes Care, 37*(2), 569–586. https://doi.org/10.2337/dc13-1203

6   O'Donnell MJ, et al INTERSTROKE investigators. Global and regional effects of potentially modifiable risk factors associated with acute stroke in 32 countries (INTERSTROKE): a case-control study. Lancet. 2016 Aug 20;388(10046):761-75. doi: 10.1016/S0140-6736(16)30506-2. Epub 2016 Jul 16. PMID: 27431356.

7   Wang, L., Shen, X., Wu, Y., & Zhang, D. (2016). Coffee and caffeine consumption and depression: A meta-analysis of observational studies. *Australian and New Zealand Journal of Psychiatry, 50*(3), 228–242. https://doi.org/10.1177/0004867415614102

8   Velickovic, K., Wayne, D., Leija, H. A. L., et al. (2019). Caffeine exposure induces browning features in adipose tissue in vitro and in vivo. *Scientific Reports, 9*, 9104. https://doi.org/10.1038/s41598-019-45540-1

9   Jing, Y., Han, G., Hu, Y., Bi, Y., Li, L., & Zhu, D. (2009). Tea consumption and risk of type 2 diabetes: A meta-analysis of cohort studies. *Journal of General Internal Medicine, 24*(5), 557–562. https://doi.org/10.1007/s11606-009-0929-5

Move as if your life depends on it

1   Song, Z., et al. (2023). Daily stair climbing, disease susceptibility, and risk of atherosclerotic cardiovascular disease: A prospective cohort study. *Atherosclerosis, 386*, 117300. https://doi.org/10.1016/j.atherosclerosis.2023.117300

2   Naci, H., & Ioannidis, J. P. A. (2013). Comparative effectiveness of exercise and drug interventions on mortality outcomes: A meta-epidemiological study. *The British Medical Journal, 347,* f5577. https://doi.org/10.1136/bmj.f5577

3   Saint-Maurice, P. F., Troiano, R. P., Bassett, D. R., Jr., Graubard, B. I., Carlson, S. A., Shiroma, E. J., Fulton, J. E., & Matthews, C. E. (2020). Association of daily step count and step intensity with mortality among US adults. *JAMA, 323*(12), 1151–1160. https://doi.org/10.1001/jama.2020.1382

4   Moore, S. C., Patel, A. V., Matthews, C. E., Berrington de Gonzalez, A., Park, Y., Katki, H. A., Linet, M. S., Weiderpass, E., Visvanathan, K., Helzlsouer, K. J., Thun, M., Gapstur, S. M., Hartge, P., & Lee, I. M. (2012). Leisure time physical activity of moderate to vigorous intensity and mortality: A large pooled cohort analysis. *PLoS Medicine, 9*(11), e1001335. https://doi.org/10.1371/journal.pmed.1001335

5   Kokkinos, P., Faselis, C., Samuel, I. B. H., Pittaras, A., Doumas, M., Murphy, R., Heimall, M. S., Sui, X., Zhang, J., & Myers, J. (2022). Cardiorespiratory fitness and mortality risk across the spectra of age, race, and sex. *Journal of the American College of Cardiology, 80*(6), 598–609. https://doi.org/10.1016/j.jacc.2022.05.030

6   Cooper, R., Strand, B. H., Hardy, R., Patel, K. V., & Kuh, D. (2014). Physical capability in mid-life and survival over 13 years of follow-up: British birth cohort study. *The British Medical Journal, 348,* g2219. https://doi.org/10.1136/bmj.g2219

7   Merom, D., et al. (2016). Dancing participation and cardiovascular disease mortality. *American Journal of Preventive Medicine, 50*(6), 756–760. https://doi.org/10.1016/j.amepre.2015.12.007

8   Verghese, J., Lipton, R. B., Katz, M. J., Hall, C. B., Derby, C. A., Kuslansky, G., Ambrose, A. F., Sliwinski, M., & Buschke, H. (2003). Leisure activities and the risk of dementia in the elderly. *New England Journal of Medicine, 348*(25), 2508–2516. https://doi.org/10.1056/NEJMoa022252

9   Song, Z., et al. (2023). Daily stair climbing, disease
    susceptibility, and risk of atherosclerotic cardiovascular disease:
    A prospective cohort study. *Atherosclerosis, 386*, 117300.
    https://doi.org/10.1016/j.atherosclerosis.2023.117300

Be stronger to live better for longer

1   National Institutes of Health. (2016, March). World's
    older population grows dramatically: NIH-funded Census
    Bureau report offers details of global aging phenomenon.
    https://www.nih.gov/news-events/news-releases/
    worlds-older-population-grows-dramatically

2   Bennie, J. A., Pedisic, Z., van Uffelen, J. G. Z., Charity, M. J.,
    Harvey, S. B., Banting, L. K., & Biddle, S. J. H. (2018). Muscle-
    strengthening exercise among 397,423 U.S. adults: Prevalence,
    correlates, and associations with health conditions. *American
    Journal of Preventive Medicine, 55*(6), 864–874. https://doi.
    org/10.1016/j.amepre.2018.07.022

3   American Heart Association. (2022, March). Resistance exercise
    may be superior to aerobic exercise for getting better ZZZs.
    *American Heart Association Epidemiology, Prevention, Lifestyle
    & Cardiometabolic Health Conference, Presentation 38.* https://
    newsroom.heart.org/news/resistance-exercise-may-be-superior-
    to-aerobic-exercise-for-getting-better-zzzs

4   Momma, H., Kawakami, R., Honda, T., Sawada, S. S.,
    Imamura, F., & Miyachi, M. (2022). Muscle-strengthening
    activities are associated with lower risk and mortality in major
    non-communicable diseases: A systematic review and meta-
    analysis of cohort studies. *British Journal of Sports Medicine,
    56*(13), 755–763. https://doi.org/10.1136/bjsports-2021-104087

5   Wang, Y., Lee, D. C., Brellenthin, A. G., Sui, X., & Blair, S. N.
    (2019). Association of muscular strength and incidence of type
    2 diabetes. *Mayo Clinic Proceedings, 94*(4), 643–651. https://doi.
    org/10.1016/j.mayocp.2018.11.031

6   Hong, A. R., & Kim, S. W. (2018). Effects of resistance exercise on bone health. *Endocrinology and Metabolism, 33*(4), 435–444. https://doi.org/10.3803/EnM.2018.33.4.435

7   Barahona-Fuentes, G., Huerta Ojeda, Á., & Chirosa-Ríos, L. (2021). Effects of Training with Different Modes of Strength Intervention on Psychosocial Disorders in Adolescents: A Systematic Review and Meta-Analysis. *International journal of environmental research and public health, 18*(18), 9477. https://doi.org/10.3390/ijerph18189477

8   Gordon, B. R., McDowell, C. P., Hallgren, M., Meyer, J. D., Lyons, M., & Herring, M. P. (2018). Association of efficacy of resistance exercise training with depressive symptoms: Meta-analysis and meta-regression analysis of randomized clinical trials. *JAMA Psychiatry, 75*(6), 566–576. https://doi.org/10.1001/jamapsychiatry.2018.0577

9   Peterson, M. D., Collins, S., Meier, H. C. S., Brahmsteadt, A., & Faul, J. D. (2023). Grip strength is inversely associated with DNA methylation age acceleration. *Journal of Cachexia, Sarcopenia and Muscle, 14*(1), 108–115. https://doi.org/10.1002/jcsm.13095

10 Labott, B. K., Bucht, H., Morat, M., Morat, T., & Donath, L. (2019). Effects of exercise training on handgrip strength in older adults: A meta-analytical review. *Gerontology, 65*(6), 686–698. https://doi.org/10.1159/000502534

Sleep soundly

1   Kripke, D. F. (2016). Hypnotic drug risks of mortality, infection, depression, and cancer: but lack of benefit. *F1000Research, 5*, 918. https://doi.org/10.12688/f1000research.8729.3

2   The European Insomnia Guideline: An update on the diagnosis and treatment of insomnia. (2023, November 28). *Journal of Sleep Research, 32*(6).

Let your lifestyle be your medicine

1   Ajay, V. S., & Prabhakaran, D. (2010). Coronary heart disease in Indians: Implications of the INTERHEART study. *The Indian Journal of Medical Research, 132*(5), 561–566.

2   Diabetes Prevention Program (DPP) Research Group. (2002). The Diabetes Prevention Program (DPP): Description of lifestyle intervention. *Diabetes Care, 25*(12), 2165–2171.

3   Morton, D. P. (2018). Combining lifestyle medicine and positive psychology to improve mental health and emotional well-being. *American Journal of Lifestyle Medicine, 12*(5), 370–374. https://doi.org/10.1177/1559827617750345

Your Emotional Wellbeing

Count your blessings

1   Emmons, R. A., & McCullough, M. E. (2003). Counting blessings versus burdens: An experimental investigation of gratitude and subjective well-being in daily life. *Journal of Personality and Social Psychology, 84*(2), 377–389.

2   Fox, G. R., Kaplan, J., Damasio, H., & Damasio, A. (2015). Neural correlates of gratitude. *Frontiers in Psychology, 6*, Article 1491. https://doi.org/10.3389/fpsyg.2015.01491

3   Emmons, R. (2010, November). Why gratitude is good. *The Greater Good Science Center at the University of California, Berkeley*. https://greatergood.berkeley.edu/article/item/why_gratitude_is_good

4   Bohlmeijer, E. T., Kraiss, J. T., Watkins, P., & Schotanus-Dijkstra, M. (2021). Promoting gratitude as a resource for sustainable mental health: Results of a 3-armed randomized controlled trial up to 6 months follow-up. *Journal of Happiness Studies, 22*, 1011–1032. https://doi.org/10.1007/s10902-020-00271-8

Give back and help others

1   Science of Generosity Project. (2024). What is generosity? *University of Notre Dame.* https://generosityresearch.nd.edu/ more-about-the-initiative/what-is-generosity/

2   Aknin, L. B., Hamlin, J. K., & Dunn, E. W. (2012). Giving leads to happiness in young children. *PloS ONE, 7*(6), e39211. https://doi.org/10.1371/journal.pone.0039211

3   Harbaugh, W. T., Mayr, U., & Burghart, D. R. (2007). Neural responses to taxation and voluntary giving reveal motives for charitable donations. *Science, 316*(5831), 1622–1625. https://doi. org/10.1126/science.1140738

4   Harding, K. (2019). *The rabbit effect: Live longer, happier, and healthier with the groundbreaking science of kindness.* Simon and Schuster.

5   Fryburg, D. A. (2022). Kindness as a stress reduction–health promotion intervention: A review of the psychobiology of caring. *American Journal of Lifestyle Medicine, 16*(1), 89–100. https://doi.org/10.1177/15598276211022299

6   Dunn, E. W., Aknin, L. B., & Norton, M. I. (2014). Prosocial spending and happiness: Using money to benefit others pays off. *Current Directions in Psychological Science, 23*(1), 41–47. https:// doi.org/10.1177/0963721413512503

7   Dunn, E. W., Aknin, L. B., & Norton, M. I. (2008). Spending money on others promotes happiness. *Science, 319*(5870), 1687– 1688. https://doi.org/10.1126/science.1150952

8   Nelson, S. K., Layous, K., Cole, S. W., & Lyubomirsky, S. (2016). Do unto others or treat yourself? The effects of prosocial and self-focused behavior on psychological flourishing. *Emotion, 16*(6), 850–861. https://doi.org/10.1037/emo0000178

9   Wheeler, J. A., Gorey, K. M., & Greenblatt, B. (1998). The beneficial effects of volunteering for older volunteers and the people they serve: A meta-analysis. *The International Journal of Aging and Human Development, 47*(1), 69–79. https://doi. org/10.2190/VUMP-XCMF-FQYU-VoJH

10 Sneed, R. S., & Cohen, S. (2013). A prospective study of volunteerism and hypertension risk in older adults. *Psychology and Aging, 28*(2), 578–586. https://doi.org/10.1037/a0032718

11 Musick, M. A., Herzog, A. R., & House, J. S. (1999). Volunteering and mortality among older adults: Findings from a national sample. *The Journals of Gerontology Series B: Psychological Sciences and Social Sciences, 54*(3), S173–S180. https://doi.org/10.1093/geronb/54B.3.S173

Stress less

1 Sapolsky, R. M. (1994). *Why zebras don't get ulcers: A guide to stress, stress-related diseases, and coping.* W.H. Freeman.

2 Almeida, D. M., Charles, S. T., Mogle, J., Drewelies, J., Aldwin, C. M., Spiro, A. III, & Gerstorf, D. (2020). Charting adult development through (historically changing) daily stress processes. *American Psychologist, 75*(4), 511–524. https://doi. org/10.1037/amp0000665

3 Segerstrom, S. C., & Miller, G. E. (2004). Psychological stress and the human immune system: A meta-analytic study of 30 years of inquiry. *Psychological Bulletin, 130*(4), 601–630. https:// doi.org/10.1037/0033-2909.130.4.601

Make time for awe

1 Sturm, V. E., Datta, S., Roy, A. R. K., Sible, I. J., Kosik, E. L., Veziris, C. R., Chow, T. E., Morris, N. A., Neuhaus, J., Kramer, J. H., Miller, B. L., Holley, S. R., & Keltner, D. (2022). Big smile, small self: Awe walks promote prosocial positive emotions in older adults. *Emotion, 22*(5), 1044–1058. https://doi.org/10.1037/emo0000976

2 Stellar, J. E., John-Henderson, N., Anderson, C. L., Gordon, A. M., McNeil, G. D., & Keltner, D. (2015). Positive affect and markers of inflammation: Discrete positive emotions predict lower levels of inflammatory cytokines. *Emotion, 15*(2), 129–133. https://doi.org/10.1037/emo0000033

3   Lopes, S., Lima, M., & Silva, K. (2020). Nature can get it out of your mind: The rumination reducing effects of contact with nature and the mediating role of awe and mood. *Journal of Environmental Psychology, 71*, Article 101489. https://doi.org/10.1016/j.jenvp.2020.101489

4   Rudd, M., Vohs, K. D., & Aaker, J. (2012). Awe expands people's perception of time, alters decision making, and enhances well-being. *Psychological Science, 23*(10), 1130–1136. https://doi.org/10.1177/0956797612438731

5   Fancourt, D., & Steptoe, A. (2019). The art of life and death: 14-year follow-up analyses of associations between arts engagement and mortality in the English Longitudinal Study of Ageing. *British Medical Journal, 367*, Article l6377. https://doi.org/10.1136/bmj.l6377

Beat burnout

1   American Psychological Association. (2023). *2023 Work in America Survey: Workplaces as engines of psychological health and well-being.* https://www.apa.org/pubs/reports/work-in-america/2023-workplace-health-well-being

2   Carr, P., & Kelly, S. (2023). Burnout in doctors practising in Ireland post COVID-19. *Irish Medical Journal, 116*(4), Article 761.

Avoid 'destination happiness'

1   Fowler, J. H., & Christakis, N. A. (2008). Dynamic spread of happiness in a large social network: Longitudinal analysis over 20 years in the Framingham Heart Study. *British Medical Journal, 337*, a2338. https://doi.org/10.1136/bmj.a2338

Learn to PAUSE

1   Kabat-Zinn, J. (2013). *Full catastrophe living.* Bantam Dell Publishing Group.

2   Hölzel, B. K., Carmody, J., Vangel, M., Congleton, C., Yerramsetti, S. M., Gard, T., & Lazar, S. W. (2011). Mindfulness practice leads to increases in regional brain gray matter density. *Psychiatry research*, *191*(1), 36–43.

3   Hölzel, B. K., Ott, U., Gard, T., Hempel, H., Weygandt, M., Morgen, K., & Vaitl, D. (2008). Investigation of mindfulness meditation practitioners with voxel-based morphometry. *Social Cognitive and Affective Neuroscience*, *3*(1), 55–61. https://doi.org/10.1093/scan/nsn004

4   Zelano, C., Jiang, H., Zhou, G., Arora, N., Schuele, S., Rosenow, J., & Gottfried, J. A. (2016). Nasal respiration entrains human limbic oscillations and modulates cognitive function. *The Journal of Neuroscience*, *36*(49), 12448–12467. https://doi.org/10.1523/JNEUROSCI.2586-16.2016

Unplug with forest therapy

1   White, M. P., Alcock, I., Grellier, J., et al. (2019). Spending at least 120 minutes a week in nature is associated with good health and wellbeing. *Scientific Reports*, *9*, 7730. https://doi.org/10.1038/s41598-019-44097-3

2   Jimenez, M. P., DeVille, N. V., Elliott, E. G., Schiff, J. E., Wilt, G. E., Hart, J. E., & James, P. (2021). Associations between nature exposure and health: A review of the evidence. *International Journal of Environmental Research and Public Health*, *18*(9), 4790. https://doi.org/10.3390/ijerph18094790

3   Stobbe, E., Sundermann, J., Ascone, L., et al. (2022). Birdsongs alleviate anxiety and paranoia in healthy participants. *Scientific Reports*, *12*, 16414. https://doi.org/10.1038/s41598-022-20756-1

4   Ferraro, D. M., et al. (2020). The phantom chorus: Birdsong boosts human well-being in protected areas. *Proceedings of the Royal Society B: Biological Sciences*, *287*(1941), 20201811. https://doi.org/10.1098/rspb.2020.1811

5   Hammoud, R., Tognin, S., Burgess, L., et al. (2022).
    Smartphone-based ecological momentary assessment reveals
    mental health benefits of birdlife. *Scientific Reports, 12*, 17589.
    https://doi.org/10.1038/s41598-022-21006-1

6   Oschman, J. L., Chevalier, G., & Brown, R. (2015). The effects
    of grounding (earthing) on inflammation, the immune response,
    wound healing, and prevention and treatment of chronic
    inflammatory and autoimmune diseases. *Journal of Inflammation
    Research, 8*, 83–96. https://doi.org/10.2147/JIR.S69656

Your Personal Fulfilment

Make every day a learning day

1   Smith, K. (2011). 'The Knowledge' enlarges your brain. *Nature*,
    479(7371), 161. https://doi.org/10.1038/479161a

2   Sarrasin, J. B., Nenciovici, L., Foisy, L. M. B., Allaire-Duquette,
    G., Riopel, M., & Masson, S. (2018). Effects of teaching the
    concept of neuroplasticity to induce a growth mindset on
    motivation, achievement, and brain activity: A meta-analysis.
    Trends in Neuroscience and Education, 12, 22–31. https://doi.
    org/10.1016/j.tine.2018.07.003

3   Snowdon, D. A., & Nun Study. (2003). Healthy aging
    and dementia: Findings from the Nun Study. *Annals
    of Internal Medicine, 139*(5 Pt 2), 450–454. https://doi.
    org/10.7326/0003-4819-139-5_Part_2-200309021-00016

Commit to making memories

1   Van Boven, L., & Gilovich, T. (2003). To do or to have? That is
    the question. *Journal of Personality and Social Psychology, 85*(6),
    1193–1202. https://doi.org/10.1037/0022-3514.85.6.1193

2 Heller, A. S., Shi, T. C., Ezie, C. E. C., Reneau, T. R., Baez, L. M., Gibbons, C. J., & Hartley, C. A. (2020). Association between real-world experiential diversity and positive affect relates to hippocampal-striatal functional connectivity. *Nature Neuroscience, 23*(7), 800–804. https://doi.org/10.1038/s41593-020-0649-0

3 Brickman, P., Coates, D., & Janoff-Bulman, R. (1978). Lottery winners and accident victims: Is happiness relative? *Journal of Personality and Social Psychology*, 36(8), 917–927.

4 Bryant, F. B., & Veroff, J. (2007). *Savoring: A new model of positive experience*. Lawrence Erlbaum Associates Publishers.

5 Carter, T. J., & Gilovich, T. (2012). I am what I do, not what I have: The differential centrality of experiential and material purchases to the self. *Journal of Personality and Social Psychology*, 102(6), 1304–1317.

Find your purpose

1 Cohen, R., Bavishi, C., & Rozanski, A. (2016). Purpose in life and its relationship to all-cause mortality and cardiovascular events: A meta-analysis. *Psychosomatic Medicine*, 78(2), 122–133.

2 Wrzesniewski, A., McCauley, C., Rozin, P., & Schwartz, B. (1997). Jobs, careers, and callings: People's relations to their work. *Journal of Research in Personality*, 31, 21-33.

3 Park, J., Kim, S., Lim, M., & Sohn, Y. W. (2019). Having a calling on board: Effects of calling on job satisfaction and job performance among South Korean newcomers. *Frontiers in Psychology*, 10.

4 Parola, A., Zammitti, A., & Marcionetti, J. (2023). Career calling, courage, flourishing and satisfaction with life in Italian university students. *Behavioral Sciences*, 13(4), 345.

Start a path to financial freedom

1   Thielen, P. (2023, March 14). The connection between financial well-being and mental health. *Forbes*. Retrieved from https://www.forbes.com/councils/forbesfinancecouncil/2023/03/14/the-connection-between-financial-well-being-and-mental-health/

Embrace yoga

1   Woodyard, C. (2011). Exploring the therapeutic effects of yoga and its ability to increase quality of life. *International Journal of Yoga*, 4(2), 49–54.

2   Desikachar, K., Bragdon, L., & Bossart, C. (2005). The yoga of healing: Exploring yoga's holistic model for health and well-being. *International Journal of Yoga Therapy*, 15(1), 17–39.

3   Gothe, N. P., Khan, I., Hayes, J., Erlenbach, E., & Damoiseaux, J. S. (2019). Yoga effects on brain health: A systematic review of the current literature. *Brain Plasticity*, 5(1), 105–122.

4   Streeter, C. C., Whitfield, T. H., Owen, L., Rein, T., Karri, S. K., Yakhkind, A., Perlmutter, R., Prescot, A., Renshaw, P. F., Ciraulo, D. A., & Jensen, J. E. (2010). Effects of yoga versus walking on mood, anxiety, and brain GABA levels: A randomized controlled MRS study. *Journal of Alternative and Complementary Medicine*, 16(11), 1145–1152.

5   Nongkhai, N., Poomiphak, M., Yamprasert, R., & Punsawad, C. (2021). Effects of continuous yoga on body composition in obese adolescents. *Evidence-Based Complementary and Alternative Medicine*.

Nurture your spiritual side

1   Brown, B. (2018, March 27). Defining spirituality. Retrieved from https://brenebrown.com/articles/2018/03/27/defining-spirituality/

2   McClintock, C. H., Lau, E., & Miller, L. (2016). Phenotypic
    dimensions of spirituality: Implications for mental health in
    China, India, and the United States. *Frontiers in Psychology*, 7.

3   Miller, L. (2021). *The Awakened Brain: The psychology of
    spirituality*. Penguin UK.

4   Miller, L., Wickramaratne, P., Hao, X., McClintock, C. H.,
    Pan, L., Svob, C., & Weissman, M. M. (2021). Altruism and
    "love of neighbor" offer neuroanatomical protection against
    depression. *Psychiatry Research: Neuroimaging*, 315.

5   Kendler, K. S., Liu, X.-Q., Gardner, C. O., McCullough,
    M. E., Larson, D., & Prescott, C. A. (2003). Dimensions of
    religiosity and their relationship to lifetime psychiatric and
    substance use disorders. *American Journal of Psychiatry*, 160(3),
    496–503.

6   Kendler, K. S., Gardner, C. O., & Prescott, C. A. (1997).
    Religion, psychopathology, and substance use and abuse: A
    multimeasure, genetic-epidemiologic study. *American Journal of
    Psychiatry*, 154(3), 322–329. https://doi.org/10.1176/ajp.154.3.322

Think yourself younger

1   Levy, B. R., Slade, M. D., Kunkel, S. R., & Kasl, S. V. (2002).
    Longevity increased by positive self-perceptions of aging. *Journal
    of Personality and Social Psychology*, 83(2), 261–270.

2   Alexander, C. N., & Langer, E. J. (Eds.). (1990). *Higher stages
    of human development: Perspectives on adult growth*. Oxford
    University Press.

3   Levy, B. R., Pilver, C., Chung, P. H., & Slade, M. D. (2014).
    Subliminal strengthening: Improving older individuals' physical
    function over time with an implicit-age-stereotype intervention.
    Psychological Science, 25(12), 2127-2135.

4   Levy, B. R., Zonderman, A. B., Slade, M. D., & Ferrucci,
    L. (2012). Memory shaped by age stereotypes over time. *The
    Journals of Gerontology: Series B*, 67(4), 432–436.

5   Levy, B. R., Slade, M. D., Murphy, T. E., & Gill, T. M. (2012). Association between positive age stereotypes and recovery from disability in older persons. *JAMA*, 308(19), 1972–1973.

6   Crum, A. J., & Langer, E. J. (2007). Mind-set matters: Exercise and the placebo effect. *Psychological Science*, 18(2), 165–171.

7   Bellingtier, J. A., & Neupert, S. D. (2018). Negative aging attitudes predict greater reactivity to daily stressors in older adults. *The Journals of Gerontology: Series B*, 73(7), 1155–1159.

8   Andrews, R. M., Tan, E. J., Varma, V. R., Rebok, G. W., Romani, W. A., Seeman, T. E., Gruenewald, T. L., Tanner, E. K., & Carlson, M. C. (2017). Positive aging expectations are associated with physical activity among urban-dwelling older adults. *The Gerontologist*, 57(Suppl_2), S178–S186.

Visualise your future self

1   Fernandes, M. A., Wammes, J. D., & Meade, M. E. (2018). The surprisingly powerful influence of drawing on memory. *Current Directions in Psychological Science*, 27(5), 302-308.

2   Boehm, J. K., Qureshi, F., Chen, Y., Soo, J., Umukoro, P., Hernandez, R., Lloyd-Jones, D., & Kubzansky, L. D. (2020). Optimism and cardiovascular health: Longitudinal findings from the Coronary Artery Risk Development in Young Adults (CARDIA) study. *Psychosomatic Medicine, 82*(8), 774–781. https://doi.org/10.1097/PSY.0000000000000855

Your Relationship with Self and Others

Start (and end) your day well

1   Picard, M., et al. (2018). A mitochondrial health index sensitive to mood and caregiving stress. *Biological Psychiatry*, 84(1), 9–17.

2   Hou, W. K., Lai, F. T., Ben-Ezra, M., & Goodwin, R. (2020). Regularizing daily routines for mental health during and after the COVID-19 pandemic. *Journal of Global Health*, 10(2), 020315.

Make your bed

1   Annes, C. K., Taylor, J. A., & Hallock, R. M. (2023, March 26). The effect of workspace tidiness on schoolwork performance of high school students. *Journal of Emerging Investigators 6(5), 1–5.* https://doi.org/10.59720/22-219

2   Association for Psychological Science. (2013, August 6). Tidy desk or messy desk? Each has its benefits. *Psychological Science.* Retrieved from https://www.psychologicalscience.org/news/releases/tidy-desk-or-messy-desk-each-has-its-benefits.html

3   Block, L. (2021, June). Happy National Make Your Bed Day! See our survey results. *Sleepopolis.* Retrieved from https://sleepopolis.com/news/happy-national-make-your-bed-day-see-our-survey-results/#survey

Be your own best friend

1   Butz, S., & Stahlberg, D. (2020). The relationship between self-compassion and sleep quality: An overview of a seven-year German research program. *Behavioral Sciences*, 10(3), 64.

2   Neff, K. D. (2009). The role of self-compassion in development: A healthier way to relate to oneself. *Human Development*, 52(4), 211–214.

Learn to let go

1   Chida, Y., & Steptoe, A. (2009). The association of anger and hostility with future coronary heart disease: A meta-analytic review of prospective evidence. *Journal of the American College of Cardiology*, 53(11), 936–946.

2   Ho, M., Worthington, E., Cowden, R., Bechara, A., Chen, Z., Yuliandari, E., Joynt, S., Khalanskyi, V., Korzhov, H., Kurniati, N., Rodriguez, N., Salnykova, A., Shtanko, L., Tymchenko, S., Voytenko, V., Zulkaida, A., Mathur, M., & VanderWeele, T. (2023). International REACH Forgiveness Intervention: A multi-site randomized controlled trial. *BMJ Public Health.*

3   Toussaint, L., Shields, G. S., Dorn, G., & Slavich, G. M.
     (2016). Effects of lifetime stress exposure on mental and physical
     health in young adulthood: How stress degrades and forgiveness
     protects health. *Journal of Health Psychology*, 21(6), 1004–1014.

Avoid idle gossip

1   Robbins, M. L., & Karan, A. (2020). Who gossips and how in
     everyday life? *Social Psychological and Personality Science*, 11(2),
     185–195. https://doi.org/10.1177/1948550619837000

2   Peng, X., Li, Y., Wang, P., Mo, L., & Chen, Q. (2015). The
     ugly truth: Negative gossip about celebrities and positive gossip
     about self entertain people in different ways. *Social Neuroscience*,
     10(3), 320–336.

3   Feinberg, M., Willer, R., Stellar, J., & Keltner, D. (2012). The
     virtues of gossip: Reputational information sharing as prosocial
     behavior. *Journal of Personality and Social Psychology*, 102(5),
     1015–1030.

4   Takahashi, H., Kato, M., Matsuura, M., Mobbs, D., Suhara, T.,
     & Okubo, Y. (2009). When your gain is my pain and your pain
     is my gain: Neural correlates of envy and schadenfreude. *Science*,
     323(5916), 937–939.

Have that friend you can call on, morning, noon and night

1   American Psychiatric Association. (2024, January). New APA
     poll: One in three Americans feels lonely every week. *Psychiatry.
     org*. Retrieved from https://www.psychiatry.org/news-room/
     news-releases/new-apa-poll-one-in-three-americans-feels-lonely-e

2   Cacioppo, J. T., Fowler, J. H., & Christakis, N. A. (2009).
     Alone in the crowd: The structure and spread of loneliness in a
     large social network. *Journal of Personality and Social Psychology*,
     97(6), 977–991.

3 Lee, E. E., Depp, C., Palmer, B. W., Glorioso, D., Daly, R., Liu, J., Tu, X. M., Kim, H. C., Tarr, P., Yamada, Y., & Jeste, D. V. (2019). High prevalence and adverse health effects of loneliness in community-dwelling adults across the lifespan: Role of wisdom as a protective factor. *International Psychogeriatrics*, 31(10), 1447–1462.

4 Kross, E., Berman, M. G., Mischel, W., & Wager, T. D. (2011). Social rejection shares somatosensory representations with physical pain. *Proceedings of the National Academy of Sciences*, 108(15), 937–939.

5 Lee, E. D., Cote', D., & Oltmans, D. (2017, March 27). Elderly loneliness and the broken heart. *American Journal of Cardiology*.

6 Holt-Lunstad, J., Smith, T. B., & Layton, J. B. (2010). Social relationships and mortality risk: A meta-analytic review. PLoS Medicine, 7(7), e1000316. https://doi.org/10.1371/journal. pmed.1000316

Remember, one day you will die

1 Ware, B. (2019). *Top Five Regrets of the Dying: A Life Transformed by the Dearly Departing*. Hay House.

Build a bridge to future you

1 Mogilner, C., Hershfield, H. E., & Aaker, J. (2018). Rethinking time: Implications for well-being. *Consumer Psychology Review*, 1, 41–53.